UNF#CK
EATING

Using Science to Build a Better Relationship with Food, Health, and Body Image

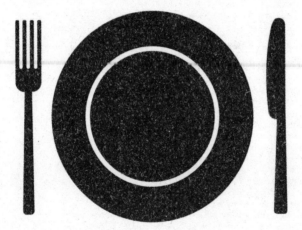

DR. FAITH HARPER, LPC-S, ACS, ACN

MICROCOSM PUBLISHING
Portland, Ore | Cleveland, Ohio

UNFUCK YOUR EATING
Using Science to Build a Better Relationship with Food, Health, and Body Image

© 2023 Faith G Harper, LPC-S, ACS, ACN
© This edition Microcosm Publishing 2023
First edition - 4,000 copies - March 28, 2023
ISBN 9781648410994
This is Microcosm #710
Edited by Elly Blue
Cover by Joe Biel
Illustrated by River Katz

To join the ranks of high-class stores that feature Microcosm titles, talk to your local rep: In the U.S. **COMO** (Atlantic), **ABRAHAM** (Midwest), **BOB BARNETT** (Texas/Louisiana/Oklahoma), **IMPRINT GROUP** (Pacific), **TURNAROUND** (Europe), **UTP/MANDA** (Canada), **NEW SOUTH** (Australia/New Zealand), **GPS** in Asia, Africa, India, South America, and other countries, or **FAIRE** in the gift trade.

For a catalog, write or visit:
Microcosm Publishing
2752 N Williams Ave.
Portland, OR 97227
https://microcosm.pub/Eating

Did you know that you can buy our books directly from us at sliding scale rates? Support a small, independent publisher and pay less than Amazon's price at **www.Microcosm.Pub**

Library of Congress Cataloging-in-Publication Data
Names: Harper, Faith G., author.
Title: Unfuck your eating : using science to build a better relationship with food, health, and body image / by Faith G. Harper.
Description: [Portland] : Microcosm Publishing, [2022] | Includes bibliographical references. | Summary: "Food is complicated. And our relationships with food and eating are all kinds of fucked up. It doesn't help that cultural messages about health, diet, body image, and weight are fatphobic and often medically dangerous. Dr. Faith Harper, author of the bestselling Unfuck Your Brain and Unfuck Your Body, brings her trademark combination of science, humor, and real talk to help us work through our food, health, and body image issues and develop a healthier relationship with food so that it can fuel us and bring us pleasure. She delves into the difference between eating disorders and disordered eating and the causes and consequences of both, breaks down the difference between various behaviors, tackles trauma and other co-occurring conditions, and provides compassionate and practical steps to improve your eating habits and repair your relationship with yourself"-- Provided by publisher.
Identifiers: LCCN 2022014754 | ISBN 9781648410994 (trade paperback)
Subjects: LCSH: Body image. | Food--Social aspects. | Food--Psychological aspects. | Eating disorders.
Classification: LCC BF697.5.B63 H37 2022 | DDC --dc23/eng/20220329
LC record available at https://lccn.loc.gov/2022014754

MICROCOSM · PUBLISHING

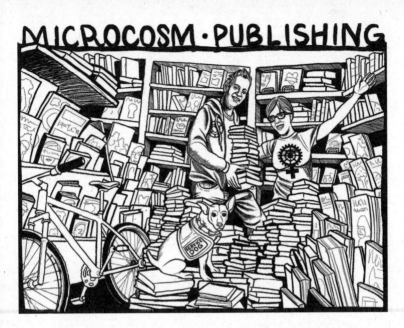

MICROCOSM PUBLISHING is Portland's most diversified publishing house and distributor with a focus on the colorful, authentic, and empowering. Our books and zines have put your power in your hands since 1996, equipping readers to make positive changes in their lives and in the world around them. Microcosm emphasizes skill-building, showing hidden histories, and fostering creativity through challenging conventional publishing wisdom with books and bookettes about DIY skills, food, bicycling, gender, self-care, and social justice. What was once a distro and record label started by Joe Biel in a drafty bedroom was determined to be *Publisher's Weekly's* fastest growing publisher of 2022 and has become among the oldest independent publishing houses in Portland, OR and Cleveland, OH. We are a politically moderate, centrist publisher in a world that has inched to the right for the past 80 years.

Global labor conditions are bad, and our roots in industrial Cleveland in the 70s and 80s made us appreciate the need to treat workers right. Therefore, our books are MADE IN THE USA

CONTENTS

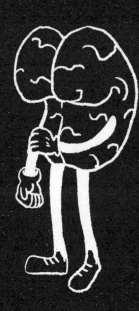

INTRODUCTION

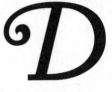**D**o you have a human body? If so, congrats, you quite probably have some issues surrounding what it looks like and how you nourish it. You definitely know someone who has struggled. Escaping the multitude of messages about how terribly wrong our bodies are (OK, maybe not Paul Rudd's . . . but mine and yours) is almost impossible. But not entirely—we *can* change our relationship with our bodies, food, and eating. Culturally, our body image ideals and ideas about food are pretty fucked. That's not our fault. But it is...I'm so sorry . . . it is our responsibility.

This book is about far more than just eating disorders and making individual, personal changes. It's about the whole disaster of modern society, capitalism, colonialism, a fucked up monoculture food system *and* disordered eating. And we need to change allllllllll of it. That feels pretty overwhelming but you aren't alone. This book is designed to serve as a toolkit for taking those first steps, no matter what point you are starting from.

So there we go, that's my goal: Humans of all shapes and sizes having normal relationships with food, their bodies, and eating again.

Again, not impossible. Difficult as hell in this society? Very.

But is it any harder than living with the misery, burden, and restrictions of constantly hating, judging, and mistreating our bodies?

I'd say not.

And when we get it right? We change the world.

What the chicken-fried fuck is "normal" eating, anyway? First of all, *normal* is just the setting on a washing machine. Not a measurable human behavior. But if we were going to take a stab at it, in terms of eating? I'd say normal would be a state of mindful consumption where one eats when hungry, enjoys food for pleasure, and incorporates a variety of foods into their diet, excluding only things that they are allergic to or truly don't enjoy. This is the opposite state from one where we eats mindlessly, or well past the point of satiation, or eats things because they are "good for them," or avoids ever eating things they really love because they are "bad for them," and never allows themselves to enjoy the social aspects of consuming food with others.

And you may be thinking, "good fucking luck being able to do all those things in this society," and you are absolutely right. I have a postdoc in clinical nutrition, and I still struggle to find a place of "normal" eating. That's why this book is for a lot more of us than one might think at first glance. While not everyone reading this may have an eating disorder, many of us have engaged in disordered eating, and most of us have struggled with disordered dieting, problems with body image, struggles with food, and diet culture, and all the other "my body isn't behaving properly for the world" nonsense that we have internalized so some fucking company can sell us some fucking product that they have convinced us will make us more acceptable, smaller, and better behaved.

And fuck all that nonsense right in the ear.

In this book, we are going to start by taking on the myths that we've been fed about how we should eat and how we should feel about our bodies. We're going to talk about body image and anti-fat bias, and the roots of all this crap in eugenics and racism and homophobia and transphobia and how much the "concern police" are actually getting wrong about health and weight (this part will be a lot of fun, trust).

Then in the second part, we're going into all the things that are listed as eating disorders in the DSM. After that, we are going to discuss those media "diagnoses." You know, the ones you see on Tiktok and the like. Orthorexia, sugar addiction, etc. What research exists, what may or may not be true about them. Fact versus fiction stuff. And there's a section at the end about diagnostic tools, for my clinical friends (and also for regular people wanting to understand how all those assessment tools work).

Presumably, you are looking for something in particular around food and eating in this book, or you wouldn't be reading this . . . but maybe not this part. People who have been fighting for their own lives against an eating disorder are often better versed in what the Diagnostic and Statistical Manual says about all of them than clinicians are. So if you are looking for more about where they all come from, skip down to the next part.

We are going to talk more in the third section of this book about what researchers know about the causes of eating disorders. Folded into that will be information about some of the people who are at higher risk than others at which point we will be discussing why some peeps are at higher risk than others. We're going to talk about how much of this is tied up in other mental health stuff. Shockingly-not-shockingly there's a lot of trauma involved, but not just that.

If you are looking for the tools to work with whatever you're dealing with, skip to part three. I start with information on the formal part of treating eating disorders but then move on to tools that you can start using right away in support of your more formal work, in regards to both your physical and emotional issues around eating and body image. Then we're also going to get into some of the tools that my clients have found the most helpful in their own work around food and body image and eating.

But seriously: Keep in mind that this is incredibly difficult work to do alone. I know people are out there rawdogging reality every day, and your survivorship is inspiring. But anyone whose eating has been disordered (and this does include perpetual dieting) for a long time has a depleted body. A professional treatment team will be beneficial if not critical to your recovery.

So I'm including some no-fee and low-fee resources for treatment as well, because I know finding care is really hard (especially if you are broke as a joke and sneak reading this in the bookstore because you can't afford the fifteen dollars rn and don't want to be the asshole who just straight up steals it, thank you for that). So when you're ready to do the work, my hope is you won't hit a brick wall of "no we can't help you unless you bring eleventy million dollars in small, unmarked bills with you." Because everyone deserves healing.

One last thing, and this is important. . . .

Food, eating, body image, body dysmorphia, diet and fitness culture . . . this can be some heavy stuff. Any particular section, or the whole book, may be too emotionally expensive for some readers to engage with right now, and it's entirely OK to know yourself well enough to skip any chapter or put this book away for the time being or forever.

If someone handed you the book and you are reading it to make them happy? Firmly close it right now and do this work when you have the energy for it. Not now if you can't. Get the support you need to take care of you properly. It's just a book and its feelings won't be hurt.

Everyone else still here? Let's get started.

Part One:

How Our Eating and Body Image Got Fucked Up

I wish there was one singular cause of disordered eating and problems with body image that I could point to so I could safely shepard everyone out of danger. Like . . . it's green socks or something fairly easily avoidable. Eating disorders are just as complex as everything else I write about, making me consider switching to writing statistics manuals instead. But here we are, yet again, trying to wrap our human brains around the complexity of massive social problems. Let's look at what the research tells us.

The biggest risk factor for an eating disorder is a history of dieting. Most diets out in the cultural ether make huge (and unsustainable) promises while being astonishingly unhealthy. People's metabolism slows down, their changes become more extreme, their starving bodies take over and they end up binging, and the constant cycling starts breaking down the body. What started out as a "I want my favorite jeans to fit again" becomes a mental and physical health crisis.

And? Most dieting doesn't start with *"I really like these jeans and they feel a little tight, I'd like to drop the 5 pounds I picked up when I started this new desk job."* Most diets start because of messaging about the wrongness of our bodies. Researchers have a lot of different phrases to describe these mechanisms like *weight stigma* and *weight teasing* and *appearance ideal internalization* and *acculturation*. But what they politely describe with this kind of phraseology is far more destructive than these phrases really allow for. Which is that *showing up simply as we are* continues to remain unacceptable in this world.

I don't think anyone exists who thinks our cultural norms around food and body image are acceptable. We have all felt that we are drowning in a sea of not-enoughness day in and day out. So it's important to really talk about that. Not just a "hahaha, fuck social media, tho, right?" way, but looking at how this feeling exists within a structure of everything we do and it's so deeply fucked up.

But before we begin, I need to state clearly and loudly the following:

Bodies come in all different shapes and sizes. They just fucking do. There isn't one ideal way for a body to be.

And this matters. Not in an effort to be supportive and empowering (though we will take that bonus content when offered), *but in an effort to be scientifically factual.* Which is why we are going to start the book with some mythbusting. What defines health? Does it have anything to do with weight? If it does, how much? Why do we prescribe to people in larger bodies, but freak out and treat in people with smaller bodies? How many trash ideas do we really have floating around in the ether?

So many, it turns out.

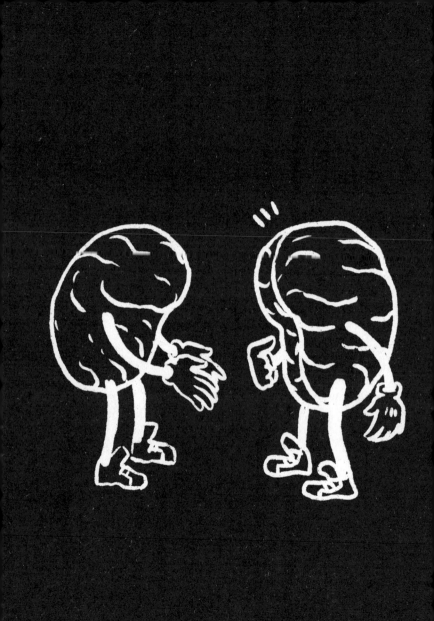

UNFUCKING WHAT WE THINK ABOUT OUR BODIES

No food is inherently bad, despite what the media will tell you.

So unless a banana cream pie actually joins the Nazi party? It's not evil. It's just food.

Calories? A source of energy. So our food (neither good or bad, just neutral) can be energy-dense or energy-light. And this energy supports many different processes in the body. A high-protein form of energy may be what you need for muscle building. A high-fat form of energy can help you absorb vitamins A, D, and E and keeps you satiated. Carbs provide energy and fuel for brain functioning. Fruits and veggies provide essential vitamins, fiber for gut health, and are correlated with many other positive health markers.

I start with this caveat because damn if the diet industry trolls us in the past few years by rebranding themselves as the "wellness" industry. And pretending these are somehow different things is like saying Meta has no relationship to Facebook and Instagram when they are actually the same damn thing with a new name tag. It's still about how your body appears to others instead of how healthy it actually is or can be. It's about wild diets that cause *literal heart damage* (per recent research sponsored by the American Heart Association), instead of promoting connection to and joy of one's own body.

But surely it has some merit if it's so pervasive right? Nah. It's pervasive because money. We've all heard about the dangers of the pharmaceutical industry's hold on western society right? The pharmaceutical industry is valued at 1 trillion (yes, a T) dollars. But the wellness industry is valued at over four times that amount. And the remaining vestiges of the diet industry are still worth billions. And just . . . ugh. I don't even know how to type out a primal scream of frustration. We're literally recommending, encouraging, and celebrating disordered eating and it really fucking has to stop.

So what is the alternative? An approach that is body-honoring instead of body-shaming. This is why programs like Health at Every Size® (HAES), Intuitive Eating, and similar others are the best frameworks to nourish our bodies and honor their differences. I'm not going to go through the principles of HAES, Intuitive Eating, or a similar model step by step. They're easy enough to find, but I do want to talk about the foundations of these movements a bit.

The goals of these models are to establish a healthy, nourishing, and joyful relationship with food. No size or weight considerations, just your ability to be embodied and joyful and engaged in your own life. What does that look like?

1) Weight loss is not the goal. It may be a side effect of adjusting to healthier habits, but it also may not. You may gain weight. It will likely just stay the same. But we're working to not care about those numbers anymore so whatever, right?

2) Once we start honoring ourselves and others within the bodies we have at the moment, we stop misdiagnosing and mistreating individuals based on our eyeball evaluation of what their bodies look like. We reduce the chances of creating more disordered eating and, frankly, we are just honoring the civil rights of all humans.

3) We are focusing on embodiment above all else. Embodiment, as expressed by self-regulation researcher Dr. Catherine Cook-Cottone, is the process of recognizing that bodies are not

something we *have,* but are instead something we *are.* Once we stop treating our body as something we have to carry around that continues to betray our desires and cause us grief, we start to heal. Once we stop measuring ourselves against the currency of what is considered desirable by larger society, we begin to heal. We become attuned to our bodies' true needs and can recognize both hunger and satiety.

4) We focus on movement as a source of play and joy, not a punitive response to what we look like or what we ate on any certain day.

5) We account for the tentacles of structural inequality in society. It recognizes the deep work we need to do as a culture to eradicate racism, transphobia, heterosexism, ableism, and everything else that walks side-by-side with anti-fat bias. Researchers Niva Piran and Tanya Luanne Teall's developmental theory of embodiment points out the need for physical freedom, mental freedom, and social power in order to remain centered in our own lives. Change isn't just individual, but it instead includes mutual aid in dismantling that which perpetuated harm against us in the first place.

These all seem like goals we should readily agree on. The sky is blue, and being mean is bad, right? So why are these extraordinary sensical goals so hard to achieve? So much of it has to do with deeply-rooted cultural messaging that surrounds class, race, and gender. And even then, maybe not in the ways you expect.

The Racist Origins of Fatphobia

Centuries ago in Europe, being full-figured was synonymous with being healthy and strong (look at Renaissance art if you want to see the ideal). This carried over to the early days of colonization of Turtle Island (now North and South America).

Because they had enough food available, American colonists weren't just heartier, they were much taller than their families back in famine-stricken Europe. By the mid 1800s, there was an eight centimeter high discrepancy between Americans and Europeans. Bigger bodies were considered more beautiful. It was fashionable for women to drink down "weight gain" tonics to catch a good husband.

The widespread trade of enslaved people was happening at the same time, and this presented a problem for those enslaving them. In order to mentally justify the ownership of some bodies by other bodies, there had to be a mechanism for deciding superiority and inferiority. This was easy at first because of skin tone. But continual rape by enslavers and interbreeding with enslaved Indigenous peoples (yes, that happened, too) meant that future generations had lighter and lighter skin. So the comparison of body types, frame size, and where fat settles on the body became the mechanism for deciding who is superior (see Sabrina Strings's amazing book *Fearing the Black Body*). White women of a certain class were able to differentiate themselves from enslaved women and poor white women by showing that they didn't have to be solid and strong to get through a day and could instead center thinness as an ideal.

Towards this new, upper crust goal of thinness, the Presbyterian minister Sylvester Graham (yes, the graham cracker guy) promoted an extremely restrictive lifestyle and diet (the original graham crackers were not yummy, trust). He died in 1851, but his followers remained active through the 1880s.

Lulu Hunt Peters, a young woman who had struggled with "baby fat" into adulthood, earned her MD and translated nutrition research to the public in what became a bestselling book. *Diet and Health: With Key to the Calories* was released in 1918 and included an extensive list of "100 calorie snacks." Dietary restrictions became the rage. Tonics meant to put on weight were replaced with ones meant to melt it away.

But then the question became, how do we decide what determines an acceptable amount of thin?

The Problem with the BMI

Today, one of the primary ways we talk about body weight and size is through the BMI. That's short for Body Mass Index, and it's the defining metric modern medicine uses to determine if your weight is healthy. The BMI was invented in the 1800s by Adolphe Quetelet, who was not a physician, but a Belgian academic who was super fired up on astronomy, sociology, math, and statistics. He was part of his era's boom in racist "science"—he is also credited with founding the field of anthropometry, which includes all that phrenology bullshit.

He was looking for ways to identify the characteristics of "the average man," thinking that represented the social ideal of manliness. He believed that someone whose physiology fit the mathematical mean of all people (which for him meant European people, but okay) would be the human ideal, which is bullshit. Based on measurements of French and Scottish men, he came up with a formula known as Quetelet's Index, which ranked his study subjects body size on a curve. It was intended as a social tool; he never meant it as a measure of body fat, build, or individual health. By the early 1900s, this index became a mechanism for determining if someone was fit to parent and as a justification for forced sterilization, also known as eugenics. It was used not just against people of color, but also poor people, people with disabilities, and neurodiverse people.

But then, capitalism. In the US, life insurance companies began compiling tables of height and weight to determine what to charge policy holders. The tables were based on the people who could actually afford to purchase life insurance and had the legal means to do so. And the numbers were self-reported. Most tables did not factor in frame size or age. And all this information was put together by sales agents and actuaries, not medical professionals.

Yet, physicians began using these unscientific tables as a means of evaluating a patient's weight as an indicator of their health. This went on through the 1950s and 60s, until medical science decided to find a more effective measure in the 70s. A research team led by Ancel Keys in 1972 conducted a study of 7,500 men (yes, only men) from five (yes, only five) different countries, trying to find the most effective measure of body fat that would be easy and cost effective to calculate during a regular doctor's office visit. They looked at those life insurance tables that doctors were using, Quetelet's Index, and other methods like the use of skin calipers and water displacement and found that all were weak but Quetelet's Index sucked the least. So the BMI remained the gold standard for measuring health.

In this study, Keys found that the BMI diagnosed "obesity"[1] accurately about 50% of the time. Meaning, that half the time individuals are carrying extra weight on their frames, and the other half of the time they just have bigger frames or a lot of dense muscle tissue. This level of "accuracy" has continued to hold at 50% (as recently as 2011, a study in the Journal of Obstetrics and Gynecology stated that, yup, it was right half the time). Can you imagine doing surgery and chemotherapy because you had a 50/50 chance of having cancer? I imagine I would be screaming my head off that they better find-the-fuck-out what's actually going on before making those kinds of decisions about my body. But if we are talking about the size of bodies and what that means about health? We decided "meh, good enough." In 1985, the National

---

1 According to the modern scale, if a BMI is less than 18.5, it falls within the underweight range, 18.5 to <25, is "normal," 25.0 to <30 is overweight, 30.0 or higher is obese, and 40.0 or higher is morbidly obese.

Institutes of Health (NIH) redefined obesity in terms of BMI. And that made it literal public policy.

The NIH wasn't done with us though. In 1998, they changed the definitions of both "obese" and "overweight," lowering the threshold of what is medically considered fat. All of a sudden, millions of people became medically (and legally) fat without gaining a pound. And now we can have a good old fashioned public health crisis over our so-called obesity epidemic and blame someone's weight for all of their medical issues.

The fallout has been all too real. There are sex based differences that are not accounted for in the BMI—which was developed measuring only white men, remember? But any woman who has ever been heavy at some point in their life has a story of being told by a doctor that their chief complaint will be resolved through weight loss.

And according to the World Health Organization, the BMI overestimates fatness and health risks for Black people while underestimating health risks for Asian communities. Many trans individuals are denied surgical gender confirmation interventions until they lose weight, even though an 18 year longitudinal study of post-op complications shows this is not necessary.

So now we have a systemic problem that disproportionately affects women, individuals of color, and trans people. People are being dismissed, other real illnesses are not being diagnosed and treated, and denied life saving treatments and surgeries based on a two hundred year old tool designed to legitimize ethnic cleansing and cultural genocide.

And I don't think the irony is lost on any of us right now.

Fat Does Not Equal Unhealthy

You can have a low BMI and not be at all healthy. Not just if you have an illness or an eating disorder—some people seem to have these insane metabolisms that keep them slim, yet they are not any healthier, or are even far less healthy, than their thicker counterparts. Over 50 studies have shown that being actually underweight (BMI less than 18.5) is associated with early death more often than being overweight.

I hit the underweight mark some years ago when my iron levels crashed out. I was sick, I felt awful, and I was shaking with cold all the time, but the number of people who told me "OMG you are so tiny! You look amazing! You are so cute!" was freakishly high. When I got treatment and was back at my healthy weight and people commented on *that*, I loved saying "Right? Thank Buddha,

I feel so much better now!" A friend of mine was bluntly told by her doctor when approaching 40, "Yes, you are tall and slim, but that doesn't mean you aren't rotting on the inside. You gotta take better care of yourself."

A "normal" BMI does not indicate health. Not even metabolically. It's so common to be in the normal or underweight BMI categories and still have metabolic issues, that there is even a term for it: T *metabolically unhealthy non-obese (MUHNO)*. MUHNO individuals may be eating like crap and not moving their body and can therefore still be insulin resistant and have high triglycerides, high blood pressure, cardiac issues, and high inflammation markers (an indicator we keep returning to again and again). Their body fat patterns are just different, not better. Extreme bodybuilding can also lead to metabolic shut down. I'm not dissing bodybuilding (my son is a weightlifter and it's a huge part of his wellness routine), but all extremes put pressure on our bodies that they aren't equipped to handle, no matter how much we would like to hack the process and live forever.

And yes, that means the opposite is also true. You can have a higher BMI and still be hella healthy. Adipocytes, the fat cells that live in our connective tissue, play a huge role in protecting us from cancer and the aforementioned metabolic diseases. Our fat also protects our bone density and is correlated with *less* risk of premature death. As a middle-aged lady who spends a lot of time talking to other middle-aged ladies I can tell you that the fluff we take on gives us cushion if (when) we fall . . . making it far less likely for us to break a hip, for example. And carrying fat is still a far healthier choice than starving (and thereby slowly destroying) our bodies. Fat can be and often is healthy. No matter how many fat cells you have (a few or a few trillion), as long as they have good circulation (which we promote with movement), we can be very, very healthy creatures.

In short? Bodies are all weird and different and each one has its own operating instructions. We can't do a little height and weight algebra equation to know if someone is healthy or not.

But one thing we do know? *The greatest indicator of life span is not your mass, it's your class.* If I wanted a good test of whether or not you are in good health and will live a long life, I would not look at your BMI or your body shape or size, but at your socioeconomic status. This is true for virtually every disease in every industrialized country. And the greater the level of inequality in a country, the greater the health disparities. Your access to care changes, the respect you are given when you do access care changes, and your access to a healthy environment and nutritious food changes.

It's Not About Willpower

We don't generally gain weight indefinitely without great determination and consequences and we also can't lose weight indefinitely without great determination and consequences. Our genetics (inherited gene characteristics) and epigenetics (how those characteristics express or not) are primarily responsible for where our bodies land in size and shape among all the other bodies out there. "Set points" are ranges of weight that your body tends to stay in, often for years if nothing else goes wrong. If you read diet books you'll find a lot of talk about "getting back to your set point" or "changing your set point" or other nonsense. In reality, *humans have three weight set points, not one.* Our weight set points are generally determined by a combination of our unique genotype, early life experiences, and epigenetics. We have our mid-point *'everything's fine'* weight, our smaller *"fit, strong, mobile, ready to avoid predation"* weight, and our large *"everything feels very destabilized, better store up some extra energy just in case"* weight. The third category seemed to get activated in an awful lot of us during the Covid-19 pandemic, btw.[2]

Another key thing to keep in mind is that *these set points are higher than they used to be.* Not just in humans but also in

---

2 Solely observational. I went up two sizes myself despite eating no differently. I've seen no studies to this effect so take it with the grain of salt with which an unsubstantiated theory should be taken.

dogs, cats, rats, mice, marmosets, etc. Again, because our set points are influenced by our environments.

Biostatistician David Allison at University of Alabama Birmingham released a report in 2010 looking at data from the 20 previous years and found that even among laboratory animals being fed incredibly strict diets, their body mass was rising significantly.[3] Science writer David Berreby, writing about Allison's research in 2013, pointed out that it clearly dethrones the false idol of individual choice. And yet, here we are a decade later, still worshipping at that same fucking altar.

Why are mammals' weights going up? Several reasons, including:

- Food itself and how it is processed today differs in how it signals insulin production

- Sleeplessness and stress (not that anyone struggles with either of these issues) affects leptin, which impacts our sense of satiety (meaning, whether or not we feel full when we have satisfied our cellular hunger)

- Viruses (scientists think a virus called Adenovirus-36 looks particularly sus in terms of weight gain)

---

3 Like lab mice were gaining 11% more body weight per decade and lab chimps were gaining 35% more weight per decade . . . with zero dietary changes.

- Bacteria (the one scientists are really watching here has a much more punk-band name to try out . . . it's called Moethanobrevibacter smithii.... and I swear my cat did not just walk across the keyboard)

- Industrial Chemicals (bisphenol-A [BPA] and organotins are frequently implicated

- Heating and Cooling (besides the biochemical influence of having electric or gas modulating the temperature we also do not have our food intake influenced by sweating or shivering from outside temperatures

- More exposure to light every day (besides the biochemical influence of the light we create, we also no longer experience normal night/day light cycles)

- Epigenetic trauma (of course I was going to include trauma! Individuals, especially if their parents went through famine while pregnant with them, will hold more stored energy as children and adults . . . the babies gestated during Holland's Hunger Winter are a good example of this phenomenon)

- Expense! A meta-analysis of studies completed by Harvard School of Public Health (HSPH) compared the prices of ultra processed foods to less-processed foods. The healthiest diets cost about $1.50 more per day than the least healthy diets, which is not as big a gap as other reports have made it seem, but still adds up to hundreds of dollars per year per person

So are we on the same page? BMI has nothing to do with health, being underweight is actually unhealthier than being overweight, having a larger body is the norm, and dieting and eating disorders will not make your body look perfect. At least not in a sustainable capacity. And not only that? They can literally kill you.

Armed with this perspective and information, let's dive into all the specific ways we can get into trouble around food, eating, and body image.

Part Two:

Disordered Eating and Eating Disorders

So what actually are eating and dieting disorders? What is body dysmorphia and how is that different? What even defines problematic body image issues? There is a lot of misinformation about this out there.

Eating disorders are adaptations created to give us a sense of control over a life that feels out of control. They're the only coping skill available to many people, and they are one that you can present for years on end without leaving the society we live in. You can still get up in the morning. You can cook, clean, caretake, work out. Go to school or work or both. Feed the dog, pick up groceries, take your elderly neighbor to the pharmacy. You can be dying inside and do and do and do and do with no one being the wiser.

We tend to think of eating disorders as the domain of cis, white women and girls. If you think about the images associated with eating disorders, the visibly underweight, light-skinned, sad-looking teenage girl is predominant. Eating disorders, feeding disorders,[4] disordered eating, body image issues affect . . . everyone. Or most everyone.

I can think of exactly one person I know who is totally content with her body. You may also know "that one

---

4 Slight difference here. Feeding disorders aren't typically about changing the shape or weight of one's body. These stem from struggles with getting enough nutrition are related to mental health issues, like sensory issues.

person," but the rest of us have bumped into issues around food and our bodies at some point in our lives.

This chapter lays out all the eating and body image issues that appear in the Diagnostic and Statistical Manual (currently in the DSM-5-TR) which is used by clinicians to assign diagnosis. Plus a bonus few that are researched and considered for future inclusion. This chapter isn't here so you can diagnose yourself, but is a tool to help figure out what to bring up with your doctor or therapist and maybe break through some of the dumb shit and misinfo you've heard over the years.

DISORDERED EATING

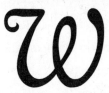e defined normal eating in the intro of this book: a state of mindful consumption where one eats when hungry, enjoys food for pleasure, and incorporates a variety of foods into their diet, excluding only things that they are allergic to or truly don't enjoy. This implies that disordered eating would be everything that falls outside the boundaries of that definition. That's a pretty universal statement, so I'm gonna do my best to de-vague-ify what I mean by that.

And, as someone who just yesterday picked a pretzel off the floor and put it in my damn mouth with all the mindfulness of a rusty shovel can tell you, almost all of us struggle with normal eating. Society isn't built for that. It's built to fuck us up about everything so it can sell us expensive solutions that don't work so we keep buying more solutions and continue to feel bad about ourselves and our bodies.

Why, after so many years of working so hard to better understand myself and my appetites and make peace with my body did I eat a pretzel from the floor? Internalized messages about not wasting food, prolly. Didn't think about it. I just ate the damn pretzel my husband dropped. No, I wasn't hungry at the time either.

So while normal is always my goal (and likely yours, too) it's a tough target to hit all the time in a rigged system. It's a continuous work-in-progress. Which doesn't mean that we are automatically failing. Liking to eat the same thing for breakfast every day, or having a propensity to stress eat more than you'd care to admit, or feeling the need to skip breakfast or work out an extra hour because you had dessert the night before, or catching yourself labeling some foods as "bad" and others as "good," or freaking the fuck out about labels in general, despite having no medical or ethical reason for needing to deep dive the ingredient list, are behaviors to pay attention to (and how to pay attention to them will be something we cover in the third part of this book). These are habits, reinforced by our larger culture, that don't necessarily interfere with our lives at this level.

So when does it become disordered eating? And when does it officially classify as an eating disorder? Like most everything else we discuss in the mental health domain, it's a matter of degree. Or rather, impact on life domain.

Using regular words instead of therapist-y words, it means paying attention to how much it's fucking up your life. It's about how your behavior around food (and burning off the calories from food) are escalating and how much all of the thoughts around food (obsessing with or or avoiding it) become invasive and all-consuming.

We say "impact to life domains" because disordered eating messes with our physical health and energy levels, as well as our ability to focus, go out with friends, hang out with family, and even sit down for a meal.

So at one end of the disordered eating spectrum, we have emotional eating, a habitual form of stuffing emotions instead of feeling them. This doesn't necessarily lead to a ton of more dangerous behaviors but often does over time. I write a lot more about emotional eating in Part 4, if you're curious. At the other end of the spectrum, disordered eating may amount to a subclinical eating disorder, or a full fledged eating disorder that just hasn't been diagnosed yet.[5] And you can be in different places on that spectrum at different times. Essentially, if you feel like something is off with your eating habits and your

---

5 It is also important to note that other researchers have found that subclinical disordered eating behaviors (which they defined as binge eating, purging, laxative abuse, and fasting for the specific goal of weight loss) are as common among cis men as they are cis women.

feelings about food, it's worth checking in about it with a professional.

Subclinical disordered eating may not have life-threatening consequences in the immediate future, but shouldn't be treated as something that will just go away with time. Even milder problematic behaviors are creating nutritional deficits and psychological distress that will only continue to impact your overall wellness . . . and likely will turn into a full eating disorder in the future.

DSM EATING DISORDERS

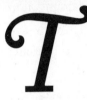hese are official diagnoses, as endorsed by the Diagnostic and Statistical Manual (as of this writing, now versioned as the DSM-5-TR). They are in this book in the same sequence they appear in the manual, so if you are a clinician or student you can use this book as a side-by-side guide. For each one, I'll talk a bit about what it entails, how it's typically diagnosed, which individuals are more likely to present with these diagnoses, and some of the most common treatment options.

Pica

Pica is an eating disorder that involves eating items that are not typically thought of as food and that do not contain significant nutritional value, such as hair, dirt, and paint chips. It isn't diagnosed in little kids, who put everything in their mouths. And it's also not diagnosed unless the things being eaten can cause a medical risk. So the 11 year old who chews on paper during class probably wouldn't be diagnosed with pica.

This also doesn't include cultural-bound behaviors. For example, the practice of eating clay has been seen in many cultures as a way of getting minerals in the diet, assisting with nausea, binding toxins in the digestive tract, a treatment for cholera and bacterial infection, and as religious practice. Kaolinite, found in soil, was so commonly used to treat diarrhea that kaolin was an active ingredient in Kaopectate until 2004.

While the numbers of people being treated for pica have increased substantially in the past twenty(ish) years, according to an Agency for Healthcare Research and Quality report, it is still considered an unrecognized and underreported disease, so the number of people living with it is generally unknown.

Pica, especially in adults, is generally related to some level of malnutrition, iron-deficient anemia being a big one. In these cases, correcting the nutritional deficiencies is generally sufficient to treat the condition. It's also common with other mental health issues like thought disorders or injuries like traumatic brain injuries, in which the brain gets confused about what is food and what isn't . . . basically anything that interferes with semantic (long term) memories. Since it's a functional memory issue, limiting the individual's access to non-food items that could be swallowed and rewarding safer behaviors (avoiding non-nutritive substances and eating nutritive ones) is the best course of treatment.

Rumination Disorder

Rumination disorder is when someone regurgitates their food regularly over a period of at least once month. It has to happen fairly regularly, at least a few times a week, and generally occurs daily. The food may be spit out when it occurs, or rechewed and swallowed. It can't be related to another eating disorder (such as bulimia) or another medical issue (such as reflux). Researchers hypothesize that it is likely an acquired habit, possibly related to the discomfort of the abdominal pressure that occurs when we eat. The regurgitation relieves that pressure, therefore actually feels good, not bad, to the person who is ruminating their food. Like with pica, the number of people who have it is underestimated and underreported. It is often mistaken for medical issues like reflux or GERD and only with time and medical testing, are we able to differentiate out that there is not a physical cause.

When it occurs in infants, it is generally related to a lack of an emotional parent-child bond. In adults, it is often related to issues with semantic memory, same as pica. The main line treatment for rumination disorder is breathing and mindfulness techniques that relax the diaphragm and help build awareness of when food is about to come up, so the body's pressure for it to come up can be managed so it can stay down. (There's an exercise for this in part four of this book.)

Avoidant/Restrictive Food Intake Disorder (ARFID)

Prior to the DSM-5, ARFID was known as Selective Eating Disorder. It still remains listed as a feeding disorder, but we have a better handle on the complexity of the disease than we used to have. While lots of people are "picky eaters," individuals with ARFID must also display either significant weight loss (or lack of expected weight gain or growth in children), significant nutritional deficiency, a requirement of nutritional supplementation (like a feeding tube or a medical meal supplement like Ensure), or significant difficulties with life domain functioning (like you struggle with work or school or going out with people because of your limitations around food).

ARFID cannot be related to cultural practices (like not eating groups of food for religious reasons), or based on limited food availability or limiting intake to change the shape of one's body (as with other eating disorders).

ARFID is most common among people with sensory issues, neurodivergence diagnoses, anxiety disorders, and a trauma history. Treatment includes helping work with any of the underlying mental health issues that may be contributing factors, finding nutrient-rich foods that are tolerable for intake, and using supplemental nutrition to address medical issues caused by nutritional deficiencies.

Anorexia Nervosa

Anorexia nervosa is known for its significant restriction of calories and resulting body weight loss as well as the individual's intense fear of getting fat, even when existing at a very low weight. Individuals with anorexia generally do not experience their body the same way that others do and/or do not see their condition as being as medically serious as it is. The severity of the disease is generally assessed based on the BMI percentile of the individual, but if other symptoms are really severe, there is a little wiggle room on the BMI component.

There are two subtypes of anorexia. The first, and by far the most prevalent, is the restricting type, which is what we typically think of with anorexia. Meaning someone who diets/fasts/or exercises excessively to burn off their caloric intake.

The second is the binge eating/purging type. This is less common, but worth getting into because it can easily be confused with bulimia, even among treatment professionals. Like bulimia, it involves binge eating and/or purging behavior (self-induced vomiting or the misuse of medications to induce moving food and fluids through the body quickly (diuretics, laxatives, enemas).

To understand the difference between binging/ purging type anorexia and bulimia, keep in mind the two types of binge eating: objective and subjective. Objective binges are when someone takes in far more than their daily caloric intake in than their body needs or they have the actual appetite for. Objective binges are a feature of bulimia, and usually involve an intake of 5000 calories or more. Subjective binges are when the amount eaten feels out of control to the person eating. So if someone used to restricting eats an apple when their intent was to not eat at all, they may feel the same loss of control as someone eating an entire bucket of extra-crispy along with all the family sized sides. So with this second type of anorexia, as the body's hunger for nutrition starts to "fight back," then we will eat what feels like a lot to us (whether it actually is or isn't) and may end up purging in a panic.

But because these standards aren't clear, some researchers and eating disorder specialists have argued that an anorexia diagnosis should be based on body weight. Meaning that even if someone is primarily binging and purging, if their body weight is as low as someone with a more traditional presentation of anorexia, that is how it is classified.

If you could see the stank face I am making as I typed that last paragraph, how much I disagree with that argument would be readily apparent. Rarely do our outsides demonstrate fully what's going on inside. Weight loss is only one of the risk factors associated with eating disorders and it isn't even the most worrisome one. So feel free to stank face along with me should you feel so inclined.

Bulimia Nervosa

Bulimia is diagnosed based on recurrent episodes of binge eating during a specific amount of time (like a one or two hour period versus snacking constantly throughout the day) followed by strategies to compensate for all the calories taken in (excessive exercise, self-induced vomiting, using medications such as laxatives, etc) to prevent or mitigate weight gain. During the binge cycles, the individual perceives themselves as out of control over their food intake and their negative self-image. If you feel out of control of your behavior, and you perceive your body negatively we experience incredible shame. We are always too much or not enough. Our us-ness isn't acceptable in its current form.

The binge-purge cycling must be occurring for at least three months, and must occur at least once a week. In fact the severity for bulimia is determined by the frequency of the binge-purge cycle in a week, which reinforces my disagreement with the diagnostic differentials between bulimia and binge-purge subtype anorexia.

Another important note in the DSM is about what constitutes an episode of binge eating. The authors of the DSM define it as "an amount of food that is definitely larger than most individuals would eat in a similar period of time under similar circumstances." Which means that Thanksgiving doesn't count here. And, on the other side of that, two pieces of pizza wouldn't either. Two pieces of pizza could feel very excessive for someone with a history of severe restriction , and they may induce vomiting because of it, but that behavior (subjective binging) would still fall under the binge-purge anorexia subtype or purging disorder, not bulimia.

Binge Eating Disorder

Binge eating disorder (BED) is the most common eating disorder in the United States.[6] It involves the eating of large quantities of food, usually very quickly and past satiety, generally to the point of discomfort. As with bulimia, in order to diagnose BED, occurrences are supposed to happen at least once a week for a period of at least three months. Severity is determined by the number of episodes that occur in a week.

The significant difference between BED and bulimia is the lack of compensatory strategies to manage the extra caloric energy being taken in. Feelings of distress, guilt, and shame are common after a binge episode, as is the feeling of a loss of control.

Other Specified Feeding and Eating Disorders (OSFED)

Individuals with OSFED commonly present with extremely disturbed eating habits, a distorted body image, overvaluation of body shape and weight, and an intense fear of gaining weight. It is significant enough to merit

---

6 Before the DSM-V it was listed under the category Eating Disorder – Not Otherwise Specified (EDNOS). EDNOS doesn't exist in the DSM-5 or the DSM-5-TR. The new catch-all category is Other Specified Feeding or Eating disorder (OSFED). Just in case you're getting tested on this material.

diagnosis, but the presentation doesn't fit in one of the categories designated above.

OSFED is the most common eating disorder among both adults (75.38%) and adolescents (80.97%). It is common (and often undiagnosed) in post-bariatric patients as well.

Another important phrase here to know here is *diagnostically subthreshold*. This means we are showing some symptoms of a condition, but without enough severity to call it a mental health issue. It's important that we not overdiagnose shit, right? Not every quirky little kid is neurodivergent, right? But we also can't ignore what may be going on with someone. Just like many first responders at the World Trade Center did not have PTSD in the first months after 9/11, many of them developed it over the next few years because the symptoms they did have were not taken seriously. Subthreshold eating disorder behaviors are the same in that researchers have demonstrated that fully half of the time they progress into a diagnosable eating disorder.

OSFED is the category we use when someone is displaying many of the key features of a feeding or eating disorder (and experiencing distress or life domain impact because of it), but not meeting full criteria for any of the disorders mentioned above. It basically means we have an eating disorder that doesn't present in a traditional way, and may be subthreshold to a more traditional presentation. The examples in the DSM-5 include:

- **Atypical Anorexia Nervosa:** This diagnosis is used when someone meets all the criteria for anorexia and, despite having lost a "significant" amount of weight, their weight is still normal or above normal. This is more common than you would think, even if underdiagnosed. Bodies develop strategies to fight back against starvation and will slow down metabolism to retain stored energy (weight), even when getting very little nutrition. Because most of the health risks associated with anorexia have nothing to do with the weight you sit at and have everything to do with the body not being properly nourished, some researchers have suggested that anyone who is presenting with a 5% or more loss of body mass and emotional/cognitive health issues should be screened for eating disorders.

- **Bulimia Nervosa (of low frequency and/or limited duration):** This diagnosis is used when someone meets all the criteria for bulimia nervosa but the behaviors occur less than once a week and/or have been happening for less than three months.

- **Binge Eating Disorder (of low frequency and/or limited duration):** This diagnosis is used when someone meets all the criteria for BED but the behaviors occur less than once a week and/or have been happening for less than three months.

- **Purging Disorder:** This diagnosis is used when someone uses purging behavior (vomiting, laxatives, diuretics, etc) to influence their weight or body shape. While the DSM-5 doesn't also list driven exercise (exercise for the sole purpose of burning off extra calories taken in . . . not like the person who works out an hour a day while listening to their favorite podcast but like the person who is on the treadmill for hours because they are panicked over having eaten an entire cheesecake), most clinicians would include that as a purging behavior (and research conducted since the DSM-5 was demonstrates that it is appropriate to do so). If you are thinking "how is this different from someone with anorexia who also engages in purging?" we're on the same page. This one is a tough differential diagnosis, without guidance on how to parse it out. I would consider the weight of the individual (since the traditional anorexia diagnosis is based on being underweight) as well as how often they are restricting. Some people with purging disorder will panic-fast after a purging session but don't generally restrict themselves. It's messy, I know. And the text revision of the DSM-5 that came out while I was writing this book didn't revise any text to help better parse out PD from other diagnoses.

- **Night Eating Syndrome:** This diagnosis is used when someone engages in recurrent bouts of "night eating." Meaning, they wake up from sleep and take in a large portion of their daily calories or they consume a lot more food after their already-eaten evening meal. The DSM-5 doesn't illuminate how much is a large portion, but most eating disorder programs look for half or more of someone's daily calorie consumption being after dinner/in the middle of the night. The DSM-5 cautions that this diagnosis shouldn't be used if BED better explains their intake and it should not be used if one is not fully aware of what they are doing (e.g., if they are sleepwalking and sleep eating). And I would suggest that it's also important to look at how much an individual is restricting during the day, because it could be a compensatory hunger hitting them late at night when they are too tired to continue to restrict.

Unspecified Feeding or Eating Disorder

Do catch-all categories make you nuts? This one actually makes a lot of sense. This diagnosis is used when there is *something* going on with eating or feeding that is causing problems in someone's life and/or a lot of distress. The clinician may not know enough to posit another diagnosis or may be choosing not to explicate the client's actual symptoms at that time for any number of reasons. This is the *"we don't feel like we know enough to say but there is definitely something going on that merits treatment, maybe an atypical presentation, maybe subthreshold diagnosis, not sure yet, okthxbai"* diagnostic code, not a cop-out.

POPULAR CULTURE "DIAGNOSES"

n top of what actually exists in the DSM-5 (and 5-TR) are other "cultural diagnoses." A cultural diagnosis can be one of two things.

- A real phenomenon that is being studied by researchers and clinicians for possible inclusion in a future edition of the DSM.

- A social media trend that currently has no backing or research to merit its inclusion.

So the ones we will be covering are in the first category. They've been operationalized enough that I can describe what researchers and clinicians have agreed might be an emerging eating or feeding disorder category. In each of these, there are enough truly concerning behaviors going on that, diagnosis aside, someone is definitely getting into a territory that can lead to lots of negative consequences.

The second category, social media trends, is too diffuse to unpack. Some possible realities may emerge from this category over the upcoming years that I can add to a future edition of this book, Creator willing. But social media is also full of misleading and, let's be real, often patently false information. For instance, I promise you that the length of your middle toe in comparison to your other toes says nothing diagnostic about you, other than a nod to your gene pool. Ask a blood relative about the toe gene if you're curious, but definitely don't write your will over it.

These following issues, however? If you are noticing these behaviors in yourself? It is absolutely time to get some support before it turns into a full-blown disorder.

Diabulimia (ED-DMT1, Eating Disorder-Diabetes Mellitus Type 1)

Diabulimia is a term used to describe a behavior by individuals with Type 1 Diabetes who misdose their insulin specifically as a purge mechanism. This type of diabetes is an autoimmune disease that requires intense attention paid to numbers and labels. You have to consider the components of what you are eating constantly. *What is the carb count? How is it mitigated by fats and proteins? What's my blood glucose after eating it? What are my A1cs? Did I gain weight? . . . That will change my medication management!* Diabetes is relentless and it often leads to *diabetes distress* (just being exhausted of the process and the time and energy it takes) which leads to *diabetic burnout* (where you disengage and stop trying). I'm unpacking all this because researchers believe that this diabetic burnout becomes a risk factor for diabulimia. Any time we are hyper-attentive to these kinds of body-based statistics, we become at higher risk for developing an eating disorder. This is why dieting so often leads to eating disorders.

Inappropriate Compensatory Behaviors to Avoid Weight Gain From Consuming Alcohol (ICB-WGA)—also known as Food and Alcohol Disorder (FAD) or Drunkorexia

Drunkorexia is a catch-all term for any behaviors that an individual may use to manage caloric intake so they can drink more alcohol. This can include restricting food before or after an alcohol binge, over-exercising, and/or purging (including drinking enough to intentionally vomit). The literature around this behavior focuses mostly on college students, but it is something that many people continue to engage in far past their college years. The numbers vary wildly, but a safe variance is that a good quarter to a third of drinkers have engaged in this behavior. There have been a lot of discussions about if this should be considered an eating disorder or substance use disorder, and I'm including it here because the restriction/compensation behavior is focused on body shape and weight.

And yeah, drinking that much also isn't conducive to good health but the behavior is more associated with disordered eating than overindulgence in substance use. And research around drunkorexia shows it's far more likely to lead to other eating disorders than to more extreme substance use issues.

Orthorexia

Orthorexia is an umbrella term used to describe disordered eating that is formed in service of trying to eat healthily, until acceptable foods become so limited other health problems and psychological distress occur. The term orthorexia has been around since the late 90s (that's the late 20th century for my younger readers) but has become more and more present as diets become rebranded as *clean eating*, or *lifestyle changes*, or *wellness plans*. And none of those things are bad in and of themselves, but they have been subverted to hide toxic diet culture behaviors with a more palatable label. Avoiding foods that you're allergic to or intolerant of is not a disorder. Wanting to eat healthy is not a disorder. Wanting to eat fewer ultra processed foods and more nutrient-dense, health-supportive choices isn't disordered. But when that care becomes increasingly restrictive it can look like:

- Compulsive checking of ingredient lists and nutritional labels

- An increase in concern about the health of ingredients

- Cutting out an increasing number of food groups (like all sugar, all carbs, all dairy, all meat, or all animal products with no moral, ethical, or medical reason to do so)

- An inability to eat anything but a narrow group of foods that are deemed "healthy" or "pure"

- Unusual interest in the health of what others are eating

- Spending hours per day thinking about what food might be served at upcoming events

- Showing high levels of distress when "safe" or "healthy" foods aren't available

- Obsessive following of food and "healthy lifestyle" blogs and social media accounts

- Body shape/size/weight may or may not be a consideration

Many people have been prescribed restrictive food plans by an incredibly well meaning medical provider. Trying to manage health issues through how we nourish our bodies is a first line of treatment for many practitioners who fall more under the functional medicine umbrella. Me included. I have seen people able to reduce medication use and regain far more quality of life with certain diet plans. But if someone has a history of dieting or eating disorders, restrictive eating plans are likely going to be off the table, and it's also important to pay attention to signs that we may be creating a new problem while trying to resolve the original one.

Food Addiction and Sugar Addiction

While the idea of orthorexia has been around since the 90s, the idea of food addiction has been around since the 50s (that's the *middle* of the 20th century, my young ones). Today, the concept of food addiction is another big one that you will see talked about on social media. 86% of Americans believe that certain foods have addictive qualities and 72% believe that these addictive qualities account for some cases of obesity.

Sugar is the big one we think we're addicted to. But spoiler? We're not really addicted to any kind of food, even the most delicious ones. I know!!! Not even Reese's

Cups! Yes, it is true that humans do have an evolutionary preference for sweetness and less of an off-switch when it comes to it. Sweet foods were a rarity in early human history (think like stumbling upon a bramble of ripe berries or whatever) and they are energy-dense. So we developed the ability to detect these mono- and disaccharides food sources readily and likely can eat more of them when they are available in order to store that energy for later.

So a sugar addiction would make evolutionary sense. But . . . that's not what the problem is. It turns out that it is higher fat foods, both sweet and savory, that researchers have consistently found to be the problem for people who are overeating in ways that we may consider addictive. Even if sweets are your bag, it's the ice cream and cookies, not sugar straight from the sugar jar.

And we just don't experience the physicality of tolerance and withdrawal around these foods. For a substance (or behavior) to be considered addictive, the human body has to experience tolerance and withdrawal. *Tolerance* refers to the physical effect of repeated use of a drug in which we stop getting relief from our original dose and need more of it. This is true of all kinds of substances. I need a higher dose of my asthma medication than I did 20 years ago, because that's the nature of being on asthma medications the entirety of my life. Tolerance alone doesn't equal addiction. *Withdrawal* is the other important component. It means that the body physically becomes dependent on that substance to maintain stasis. Once that substance is no longer available, we get sick. And with some substances, like alcohol and opioids, we can get so sick that we will die without medical intervention.

And food? Even something very delicious and satisfying does not invoke tolerance and withdrawal.

If certain foods are able to hijack the reward systems in our brain, blocking those reward signals would have some effect, as they do with drugs. ΔFosB (Delta FosB) is a regulatory protein in the human body that has been found to play a significant role in the development of and maintenance of chemical addiction. If your body tends to overexpress this protein, you are more likely to fall down the addiction rabbit hole. However, ΔFosB has not been connected with foods in humans. Blocking dopamine function has been tested and found to be ineffective in managing what we have termed food addiction for going on a century now. Using an opioid blocker[7] has also proven unhelpful.

Essentially, as far as researchers have found (at the time of me writing this) there is no neurobiological

---

7 This is actually an incredibly sensical test. The only non-substance addiction in the current DSM is gambling. One of the best treatments for a gambling addiction is an opioid blocker.

underpinning for food addiction based on how we understand and measure addiction. The scale used to measure food addiction, is likely measuring a subtype of binge eating disorder instead.

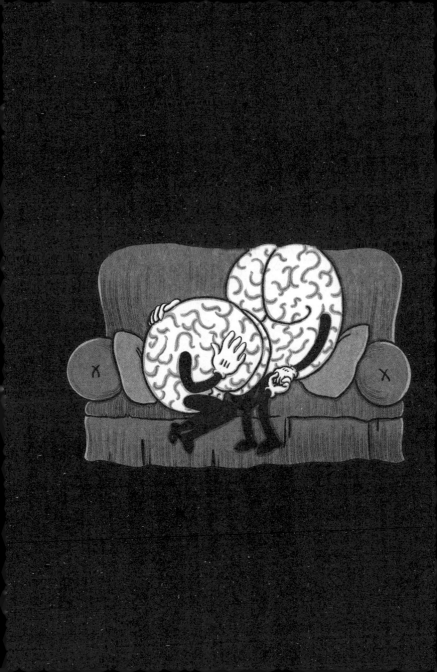

BODY DYSMORPHIA

Body dysmorphic disorder (BDD) is a disorder within which we become obsessed with minute or imaginary flaws or differences in our appearance. This one *is* in the DSM, but it isn't an eating disorder, and it isn't listed with the eating and feeding disorders. When it first appeared in the DSM, it was the DSM-III which was released in 1980, and it was listed as an atypical somatoform disorder. Which is actually a bit rude, seeing that somatoform disorders are the category that the cranky olds used as a more polite way to say, "It's all in your head, you're making shit up." Hypochondriasis? A somatoform disorder. But by the DSM-5 we got it situated more appropriately, hopefully helping clinicians better understand what is really going on.

BDD is a disease of self-perception, therefore is categorized with Obsessive Compulsive and Related

Disorders. And yes, it's really hard to be alive in this day and age and have a healthy sense of self and a clear perspective of one's body, but individuals with body dysmorphia struggle to an extreme that it causes distress and impairment in life domain functioning. There is an intense preoccupation with at least one aspect of the individual's physical appearance that they believe to be a flaw or a defect. This flaw seems huge to the person in question but is generally not even noticed by those around them. So like a tiny bump on the cartilage of one's nose becomes a monstrosity of a Cyrano nose in their mind. This "flaw" then leads to compulsive and repetitive behaviors in response to their appearance concerns. Constantly looking at aforementioned flaw in the mirror. Feeling a need to fuck with it all the time (grooming, skin picking, tanning, etc.) to minimize it, seeking surgical interventions,[8] or asking for reassurance from others exhaustingly. And if it is BDD, the flaw can't be specific to body fat or weight if there is also a concomitant eating disorder.

OK, if it isn't an eating or feeding disorder, why are we talking about it? Because we are talking about all the ways that perceptions of our bodies and how we nourish them

---

8 Because I get asked this several times a year, gender dysphoria is clearly not a form of BDD. Surgical interventions provided to someone with BDD don't help. In fact, they often make the BDD worse. And gender confirmation surgeries for someone who is not cisgender provide significant symptom relief and psychological benefit. Are we good on this yet? Great. Thanks.

are impacted by mental health. Body dysmorphia is not a bullshit *"oh, I'm not happy with my thighs when I look in the mirror"* issue, but needs to be recognized as the incredibly debilitating mental illness that it is. It is as difficult to treat as the eating disorders mentioned above and is also often experienced with other complex diagnoses (mood disorders, thought disorders, anxiety, obsessive-compulsive disorder, and even tic disorders are present in higher rates among people with BDD). Suicidality is also frighteningly common. Thoughts of suicide are experienced by 80% of individuals with body dysmorphia at some point during the course of their illness, and a quarter of individuals will make a suicide attempt. And the number of individuals with BDD who die by suicide is also extraordinarily high— 45 times higher than that of the general population.

Muscle Dysmorphia (Bigorexia)

Just like "being healthy" can lead to disordered eating, "being fit" can transmogrify into a significant mental illness. Because we associate big arms and low body fat with fitness, it is easy to assume that guys like The Rock are super healthy. But, when it overshoots to become an obsession, it has a special name, "muscle dysmorphia," or informally, "bigorexia."

Muscle dysmorphia isn't a separate diagnosis from BDD, but is actually a BDD specifier. So if someone has muscle dysmorphia, they get a BDD diagnosis with a note that it is muscle dysmorphia specifically. Aaron Sapp (Dr. Sapp, if you're nasty) and I wrote about this in our zine *Detox Your Masculinity*, and I am including it as a separate column from traditional BDD because it presents so differently.

This version of body dysmorphia is far more likely to present in men than women. Bigorexia is a fantastically useful word for it too, because it illustrates how the need to be big is just as harmful as the anorexic's need to be small. Guys who have bigorexia don't see an accurate image of themselves when they look in the mirror. Even when they look like Captain America they see Pee Wee Herman.

While bigorexia is a disorder of bodily perception, it is far more likely to involve disordered food intake as well. What is being passed off as healthy eating, really isn't. Someone with muscle dysmorphia isn't getting nearly enough of their energy from fats. They have way more protein than they need, and quite likely their gut would appreciate some damn fiber. People with this disease believe that if they consume too much fat or too many calories, they will lose muscle definition. Because it is not about what the muscles allow them to *do*, it's about what the muscles make them *look like*.

ASSESSMENT TOOLS

hat was a lot! It's entirely ok to stop, stretch, breathe, and hydrate. Everything above may have been information you were already well aware of or some of it may have been pretty new. And you may be having an "oh, shit…it me" moment. And if you are in the latter category, please don't try to do this work on your own.

We're going to look at what treatment may entail in the 4th part of this book. But the first step is to talk to your doctor, therapist, or other care provider about your concerns. You may be worried that they will dismiss your concerns, But a competent provider will assess you properly. So *this* section is for both my clinicians who want to make sure they are using the best assessment instruments and for anyone seeking treatment who wants to prepare for advocating for yourself. Let's talk about that in a clinical way while all these different criteria are fresh in our minds

One thing that you'll notice over and over in this book is that rates of eating disorders vary wildly in different studies and data collection efforts. We suck at screening effectively. This is a problem everywhere in our field, but it's really glaring when we start looking at mental health disorders that focus on eating, dieting, and body-presentation.

So whether you are a clinician or someone who is looking to better understand the field and advocate for your own care, it's important to know what assessment tools can do and not do. I looked at a hell of a lot of data on factor analysis and validation of different scales so I could recommend the best ones I could find. Additionally, all the ones I've included here are free to access and use. They are not free to republish so you have to do your own search on that little computer in your pocket, but you don't have to pay a ton of money to some big corporation to use any of these tools.

And while it shouldn't have to be said, it still often does: No singular assessment tool should be the determining factor for a diagnosis. Whether it is a basic screener or a far more intensive tool, all the data collected should be guiding the decision-making process, not hurling the decision-making process toward a brick wall. This means you aren't going to take one of these tests and be officially diagnosed—you'll also have to answer a lot of general questions and quite likely have to do some assessments for depression, anxiety and the like. It may be a cumbersome process, but it's far better than just throwing darts blindfolded.

- The SCOFF Questionnaire: This is a 5 question instrument based on the core features of anorexia and bulimia. It's an early screener, similar to how the CAGE is used as a substance use screener.

- The Eating Disorder Examination Questionnaire (EDE-Q) is a 28-item self-reported questionnaire based on the semi-structured interview format of the Eating Disorder Examination (EDE). It uses four subscales to look more closely at range and severity of restraint behaviors, eating concerns, shape concerns, and weight concerns. The EDE-Q is designed for ages 14 and up, and the adapted Eating Disorder Examination for Adolescents (EDE-A) is designed for ages 12-through adolescence. There is a shorter (12 question) version if 28 questions is more than can be tolerated that is also validated. And (but wait! There's more!) there is the EDE-Q designed for family members and caregivers.

- Nine-Item ARFID Screen (NIAS) is a nine-question likert scale designed to identify concerns around the factors of picky eating, appetite, and fear that can help identify an ARFID diagnosis

- The PARDI is a newer, structured-interview assessment developed specifically for the three feeding disorders (ARFID, pica, and rumination disorder). It continues to be studied beyond its initial reliability and validity testing, so more about its efficacy as an instrument will be forthcoming in the next few years.

- The two scales that have been found to be fairly rigorous for assessing for body dysmorphic disorder are the Body Dysmorphic Disorder Questionnaire (BDDQ) and the Dysmorphic Concern Questionnaire (DCQ). Both are fairly basic screener tools, but the BDDQ is the one you are most likely to see if you are being cleared for plastic surgery.

- For the version of body dysmorphic disorder known as muscle dysmorphia (bigorexia), the MDDI (Muscle Dysmorphic Disorder Inventory) will be more appropriate in capturing the information needed to help make a determination of this particular subtype of BDD.

Great, stats nerd. What about the other ones? The not-officially-in-the-DSM ones that may have some merit and should be watched for? I got you there, too.

- For ICB-WGA, two scales have been created. The Drunkorexia Motives and Behaviors Scale (DMBS) has th

- us far held up to analysis while the more commonly used Compensatory Eating and Behaviors in Response to Alcohol Consumption Scale (CEBRACS) has not.[9]

- For orthorexia, many people use the Bratman Scale which was designed by the individual who first coined the term. However, the scale that has been most consistently validated is the Dusseldorf Orthorexia Scale, which is now available in English as well as several other languages beyond German.

- What about whatever it is we are trying to measure around this concept of food addiction? Several tools have been found to be reliable in validly measuring something which may or may not be a true process addiction, but may be helpful to your work. The Highly Processed Food Withdrawal

9 For my research nerds? The CEBRACS is not just noninvariant, it has failed to produce confirmatory analysis of its four factor model.

Scale (ProWS) is a self-report questionnaire that assesses 29 physical withdrawal symptoms that we may experience when cutting down or cutting out ultra processed foods. It was based on prior measures related to withdrawal from THC and tobacco so it is often used as a measure of food addiction for this reason. The Anticipated Effects of Food Scale (AEFS) is another self-report scale based on expectancy theory and substance use to measure these as constructs within the consumption of highly processed versus minimally processed foods. And finally, the very well known Yale Food Addiction Scale (YFAS 2.0) is used to measure addictive behaviors around food in general (also based on substance use scales). I'm including these despite all my hesitations around food addiction as a concept at all, because I think they are still picking up important information around how we use food to soothe and cope, which may be clinically valuable. High scores on the YFAS 2.0 have also been associated with (and therefore may help diagnose) binge eating disorder, anorexia nervosa, and other possible subthreshold eating disorders.

Part Three:

What

Makes

It

Worse?

Ok, so that was deeply unfun, wasn't it? That long list of bad things we just went through? So I know you are now excited to explore what causes these issues, to the best of our knowledge?

I know, not really. *But.* . . .

This is also important. Remember how we talked in part one about the biggest risk factor for eating disorders being a history of dieting? Well, there's a *lot* more to it than that. Because there are no singular causes of eating disorders. It's a big, messy ball of correlations that help us understand why we are so susceptible.

That doesn't necessarily mean that, for example, racialized trauma was the singular trigger to your disordered eating. Or that if you have a substance use disorder you clearly also have an eating disorder. But each of these experiences or cultural touchstones add another layer of likelihood that this is something you'll have to deal with in your life.

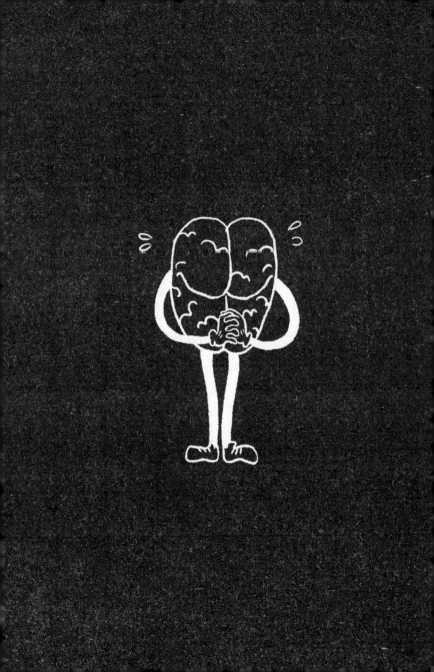

CULTURAL RISK FACTORS

Living in a Looks-Oriented Culture

Just existing within our larger looks-and-size obsessed culture is the ultimate risk factor for eating disorders. And that's all of us, at least to some extent. And as you'll see by the end of this section, the more of that culture we consume and participate in, through media and socialization, the more likely we are to develop body image problems.

Researchers disagree with each other all the time. Especially behavioral health researchers. Vehemently and with great pettiness and many multisyllabic words about most everything, but one topic most everyone is on the same page about? There are huge advantages to be had if you have a body that is considered physically attractive.

Time and again, researchers have found that people connect what we perceive as facial attractiveness to all admirable human qualities. Like intelligence, moral goodness and better interpersonal skills. Not that hotness has anything to do with any of those things. But because we do have this false equivalence? People who are considered attractive are also believed to have easier lives in general. You may feel everything around you is being held together by silly string, but if you are hot the presumption is that if you're attractive you have more happiness, more life satisfaction, a better salary, better friends and family, and are just more socially competent.

And sure as fuck do we swallow that narrative as immutable truth really early in life. If a societal ideal sticks its landing in us before we have much capacity for critical thinking, the results are staggering.

By age 6, when most everyone is in school, girls start expressing concern about their shape or weight. About half (research says 40-60%) of elementary school girls demonstrate a concern about their weight and becoming fat that they carry throughout their lives. Almost equal numbers of boys and girls (40% of overweight girls and 37% of overweight boys) are teased about their weight by peers and/or family . . . really sticking home the message that they are not compliant or acceptable. Of course, this shaming actually causes *more* weight gain, more disordered eating, and more mental health issues. The only thing it encourages *less* of? Engagement in sports and other forms of physical activity.

But man, the messages tell us to keep attempting this bodily perfection. So we do. 62.3% of teenage girls and 28.8% of teenage boys report efforts at weight loss, with 58.6% of girls and 28.2% of boys actively dieting. Half of the the teenage girls and almost a third of the teenage boys i who were already trying to lose weight are doing so in unhealthy ways Additionally, 68.4% of girls and 51% of boys exercise not for the joy of being in their bodies but with the articulated goal of losing weight or avoiding weight gain. And yet? 95% of all dieters will regain the weight they lost within five years and usually within the first year.

And before you @ me? Yes, I know that not *all* beauty standards are culturally transmitted. Studies of infants across cultures have found, time and again, that there are certain human features that we have an evolved preference for, including facial averageness (people who kinda look similar to most everyone else rather than having distinct/ strong features), symmetry (balanced features), skin homogeneity (skin tone smoothness, not color) and sexual dimorphism (pronounced visible differences between the sexes as assigned at birth).

Which, of course, leads to some fucknut on some social media platform to decide that they, as a premier Reddit "researcher," have proof of gender essentialism and the like. But keep in mind, first of all, that we have lots of evolutionary wiring that doesn't serve modern society. Everything from our physiological stress responses to the weird shape of the human penis have well-established evolutionary roots that have almost nothing to do with modern human needs and experiences. But more importantly, people have always existed in all shapes and sizes and gender fluidity . . . *but we didn't used to be such astonishing assholes about it.* So what broke us?

We have all these little cognitive shortcuts (heuristics) that our brains have developed so we can make faster decisions about the world around us. One of them is called *prevalence-induced concept change.* The idea is that what we see defines our normal. And media images specific to how bodies present may be a direct influence. So researchers designed a specific study with a true experimental research design to test the theory. Participants were shown body images flashing across the screen.[10] One group saw the same mix of body types and the other got a shifting perspective where they saw more and more of the thin bodies.

Research subjects who saw mostly thin bodies shifted their perspective on who was overweight to include bodies

10 It was like a basic, clearly computer created, body shape image of a generic light-skinned femme. So they singled out size specifically and didn't test skin color/hair/gender presentation, etc. Seeing how those moderate the effect would be a fascinating follow-up.

that were completely normal, even by our shitty BMI standards. And y'all? I looked at the computer images they used in the research. And what I mentally labeled as "small-normal" was actually underweight. Fuck, that hurt my heart.

And man, it happens fast. If you didn't grow up in traditional Western culture but become exposed to it later? You're still just as susceptible. A study of women in Fiji during the first three years after the introduction of Western television augments this point. Women who had been perfectly content with their bodies shape, size, and presentation developed serious issues around body image and eating disorders. At the three year mark, 74% of the women in the study identified themselves as "too fat." 69% had dieted to lose weight during the study time period, and 11% had started purging. Almost 30% of the women (in a study of women who felt *just-fucking-fine* about their bodies before they saw our fucked up TV media) qualified for an eating disorder diagnosis.

This particular study also nods to other considerations about what is going on here. As we established back in the first part of the book, most people in the world will never fit into a Western designed-and-reinforced model of beauty and health because everything about the model is fundamentally racist, sexist, queerphobic trash.

Sociocultural Idealization of Thinness as Anti-Fatness, Anti-Blackness, and Anti-Queerness

Yes, race is a social construct, but it's a social construct that continues to impact every aspect of our lives. Where it's been studied, the rates of eating disorders tends to be higher. Black teenagers are 50% more likely than white ones to demonstrate binge and purge behaviors. Hispanic individuals are also significantly more likely to exhibit bulimia-related behaviors than non-Hispanics. And binge eating disorder has much higher prevalence in all racialized minority groups when compared to national averages.

And race isn't the only factor that makes you more at risk of an eating disorder. Compared to other populations, gay and plurisexual men are disproportionately found to have issues with body image and engage in disordered eating. While research says that gay men are only thought to represent 5% of the total male population, they represent over 40% of the men who have eating disorders.[11] Additionally, transgender individuals experience eating disorders at significantly higher rates than cisgender people. In fact, in a recent survey of college students, transgender students were way more likely to report an

---

11 Connectedness to the larger queer community is a protective factor against disordered eating. So it's not queer culture causing the issue, it's the larger culture surrounding it.

eating disorder diagnosis than any other minority group on campus.

Yet despite minorities experiencing eating disorders in the same or, more likely, higher numbers they are far less likely to receive help, care, and support. One research team created a quite eloquent study where they presented treatment professionals with a fictional case study of a client with disordered eating. The woman in the fictional case study was presented as either white, Hispanic, or African-American. 44% of the clinicians thought the eating disorder behavior was problematic for a white woman. 41% thought so for a Hispanic woman. Only 17% did so when it was a African-American woman. In the same study, clinicians were far less likely to recommend professional care to the African-American woman.

It's not just access to care being a structural issue, but how professionals think about groups of people and their potential treatment needs. And that problem harkens back to the invention of the BMI and its continued use today.

Hegemonic Masculinity

The earliest case studies of anorexia nervosa were published by Richard Morton in 1690 and included cases of a man and a woman. Eating disorders have never been "women's diseases."

Body image issues are just as prevalent in men as they are women. But they are far less likely to be recognized and treated in men, and because of this, a larger percentage of men will die from the effects of their eating disorder. It's especially bad for men in their teens through young adulthood.

Men are far more likely to be quiet about their body image struggles, are less likely to seek treatment, and will hold off on starting treatment far more often than women because of the shame associated with their experience. We aren't saying it's easy for women to seek help. But we've made it even harder for individuals of other genders to seek help because we have learned to associate help-seeking behavior with weakness and unmanliness.

Remember Adolphe Quetelet inventing the BMI because he was trying to find the "average" or ideal male body? There is no universal checklist for what makes someone ideally masculine. Our assumptions and biases about this vary from culture to culture and within cultures over time. Just think about how different film stars from the 40s look from what we see on the screen today. Or how different business dress appears from Japan to Saudi Arabia. Heck, in lots of countries, straight men holding hands with each other is completely a thing. It can be super harmful to believe that the rules for being male you see presented in your media are the only way to look, act, or be masculine.

The term "hegemonic masculinity" has been around since the 1980s and refers to structures in place to support power and control by a very particular version of men. The five components of hegemonic masculinity are:

- Distancing yourself from anything that is associated with "femininity"

- Restricting emotions to those deemed appropriately "masculine" (like anger)

- Avoiding vulnerability

- Having others bow to your superior sexual prowess (with women)

- Utilizing homophobia to prove your heterosexuality

These characteristics make it easier to understand how body image issues appear in men and how difficult it is to even have conversations about these issues, let alone treat them.

What we see in others informs what we see in ourselves. And if what we see is skewed, then our view of ourselves is skewed.

Some facts to consider:

- Unrealistic media imagery around men's bodies is just as prevalent with men as it is women. And that's not just about weight, but also muscles, hair, and penis size to start out with.

- 95% of college-age men express body dissatisfaction, as do 90% of men in general.

- Purging and extreme dieting increased at a faster rate in men compared to women from 1998 to 2008.

- Research shows that up to 40% of individuals with eating disorders are males, but the prevalence of diagnosable eating disorders in males is likely even greater than estimated, because men are often too stigmatized to seek treatment for "women's problems" and because assessments tend to score males lower than they should.

- Men are more likely to demonstrate eating disorders that don't present in the classic hyper-restriction of anorexia or the binge and purge cycles of bulimia and concomitant substance abuse than women, which means some tests may not reflect the different ways men present with disordered eating.

Aesthetic Athletics

While all sports involve the physicality of our bodies, certain ones are more likely to focus on size, weight, appearance, and diet. Don't get me wrong, healthy participation in sports and exercise is almost always good for our health and our self-image. But some sports can come with a higher risk of eating and body image issues. People of all genders who participate in sports with a strong emphasis on aesthetics (like bodybuilding, gymnastics, swimming, and diving) and weight-classed sports (like wrestling, boxing, horse racing, and rowing) are more likely to experience disordered eating. For example, researchers in one study found that within these sports categories, 33% of male athletes and 62% of female athletes qualify for an eating disorder diagnosis, based on how they manage their body shape and weight for sports performance.

In fact, this is so common that researchers and treatment providers refer to the "Female Athlete Triad" as the combination of disordered eating, amenorrhea (the loss of menstruation), and osteoporosis (bone density loss). While this combination is seen in female athletes of all ages, it is incredibly common in adolescent girls because the body is still developing.

This is not to say that people should steer themselves and their kids away from these or any sports, but it will mean an extra eye on messaging they are getting about their bodies in the process of competing.

HEALTH RISK FACTORS

*T*he following conditions or diagnoses also often go hand-in-hand with eating disorders. Having one of these increases your chances of also having an eating disorder, disordered eating, or jacked up body image.

Trauma

What a big fucking surprise that a Dr. Faith book includes something about the impact of trauma on whatever topic I'm writing about. And guess what? A correlation between trauma history and eating disorders is definitely a thing. Especially childhood trauma and historical trauma (epigenetic, intergenerational trauma).

Childhood trauma is typically measured with the Adverse Childhood Events (ACEs) scale. It doesn't just refer to a singular traumatic event like a loss or an injury.

It can also mean growing up in an unsafe, insecure, or unsupportive environment.

The historical trauma research is emerging, and most of what is available now is focused on discrete groups like descendants of Jewish Holocaust survivors, individuals with enslaved ancestors, and individuals of Indigenous decent. These studies are finding evidence of both continued mental health issues and the physical health consequences of carrying intergenerational trauma.

You might be wondering how a traumatic event can cause something like an eating disorder, years, decades, or even generations after it's over. The short answer is that the body responds to all pain with a protective mechanism to promote healing and recovery. We call it inflammation, and it can stay upregulated for a long time in individuals with unhealed trauma. The thing about that pain response is that *your body does not distinguish between physical and emotional pain*. You read that right. The body responds to all trauma, whether getting hit by a car when crossing the street or the death of a loved one with an inflammatory response. Inflammation is the body's way of saying "slow down so we can heal." You can read more about this in my book *Unfuck Your Body*. For now, just know that inflammation is a major risk factor behind depression and anxiety, which we often try to cope with by using disordered eating as a soothing method. Which in turn can cause more inflammation, continuing the cycle.

Approximately one in four people studied for inpatient treatment for an eating disorder also had symptoms of post-traumatic stress disorder (PTSD). I'd say it's more than that...but this is also my treatment specialty so I may have a jacked perception. But either way, the researchers focused on childhood trauma found that emotional abuse was the biggest predictor of disordered eating over any other type of abuse.

Now, operationalizing emotional abuse is difficult, and bless the researchers working to do so in a rigorous manner. My best guess, from my clinical experience, is that it's tied into other research that demonstrates two other risk factors for an eating disorder:

- Anyone with a close relative (like a person you grew up with) with an eating disorder or a mental health condition presents a huge risk for the development of an eating disorder.

- Having a history of what researchers call *self-oriented perfectionism*. Meaning, the onus is not on others to perform at a certain level, but for yourself.

Anita Johnston's book *Eating in the Light of the Moon* has resonated significantly with a number of my clients, because it addresses these emotional neglect and abuse indicators of eating disorder development. She positions eating disorders as a response to being a highly attuned, empathic person growing up in a home where honesty and accountability and stability were discounted or denied. You start to distrust your responses and also need a means of coping with the distress of your surroundings . . . while still remaining relatively functional. In the last part of this book, I'm going to share how I've expanded on her model to help individuals in recovery reclaim that abandoned self.

Substance Use Disorders

According to the National Center on Addiction and Substance Abuse, up to half of individuals diagnosed with an eating disorder are also abusing alcohol or drugs. This rate may match what is happening on any college campus on any regular day, but it still is a rate that is 11 times higher than the eating disorder rate of the general population.

Most research on the co-occurrence of the two demonstrates that the eating disorder usually emerges first, and as it strengthens, it lends to the development of substance use problems. But even with this high prevalence rate, and the emergence of research that indicates the importance of ongoing screening and monitoring, very few programs provide simultaneous treatment of substance use disorders and eating disorders.

SAMHSA's National Treatment Center Study data found that of the 351 publicly funded substance abuse disorder treatment programs, only half of them screened for eating disorders (and only 14% of the ones who did used a standardized assessment), 16% offered co-occurring treatment, and a minute 3% of these programs have a formal referral arrangement with outside providers who could provide eating disorder treatment.

It doesn't help that no evidence-based practices have been established for the simultaneous treatment of both, so there are likely plenty of programs that would love to offer something but are stuck because of their funding requirements. So any of my grad student readers out there that are looking for a research project, please consider this one, we need your help.

Neurodivergence

Eating and feeding disorders are pretty frequent among people with neurodivergence diagnoses, which is to say Autism Spectrum Disorder (ASD), Attention Deficit Hyperactivity Disorder (ADHD), and Obsessive Compulsive Disorder (OCD). Researchers think the connection likely is related to executive function differences, impulsivity, and lower dopamine production.

Individuals diagnosed with ADHD are at higher risk for all eating disorders, but bulimia nervosa and BED are the most common. Additionally, as ADHD symptoms worsen, so do eating disorder symptoms when both are present.

It is also incredibly common for autists to have issues with food and eating. One study of autistic children found that 70% of those surveyed had issues with food and eating. And of course eating a restricted diet to help manage sensory overwhelm isn't a problem in and of itself. Often the disordered eating among autistic people comes with issues other than body shape and weight, making ARFID a common occurrence among autists. Even with other eating disorders, like anorexia, there is less direct correlation to body shape and weight than with other individuals with anorexia.[12] Contributing factors are thought to include:

- Sensory issues (not just around the food but also recognizing hunger signals)

- A need for specific routines and control

12 One study showed that up to 35% of the women with anorexia who were in an eating disorder program qualified for a diagnosis of Autism Spectrum Disorder.

- Social isolation
- Food or mechanisms around food become an interest/obsession or a means of managing other anxieties

And then there's OCD. With the DSM-5, we saw a big change in how OCD was thought about. It is no longer considered an anxiety disorder, and instead is recognized as a form of neurodivergence. The prevalence rates vary fairly unhelpfully but consistently show that OCD symptoms are way higher among people with eating disorders than the general population. In fact, some researchers consider eating disorders part of the OCD spectrum. Why the huge overlap? Most disordered eating involves pretty significant ritualistic compulsions in order to alleviate uncomfortable or painful emotions. Even with diseases like anorexia, there are incredibly complex rituals around not-eating, similar to what someone who binge eats may experience around eating.

Other Mental Health Issues

Eating disorders can cohabitate with any number of mental health conditions. A study of individuals hospitalized with an eating disorder found 97% of them had another co-occuring mental health condition. But certain mental health conditions are more prevalent than others.

Mood and anxiety disorders are the huge ones you will most likely see someone with an eating disorder also struggle with. Two-thirds of people with anorexia demonstrated signs of an anxiety disorder several years before their disordered eating began. In the study of hospitalized individuals, over half of the people with any eating disorder also had an anxiety disorder. Mood disorders are even more prevalent, with 94% of the individuals in the same study having a diagnosed mood disorder, most typically Major Depressive Disorder.

None of this is designed to say trauma causes eating disorders, eating disorders cause depression, or any other nonsense you see in click-bait articles. It is to say that it is really fucking hard to walk in this world. And those of us who are particularly sensitive to the fuckery around us are more susceptible to a host of issues because of it. And the presentation of one mental health issue is often only part of what is going on.

Part Four:

Unfuck Your Eating

I know that within all my books I say something to the effect of, "Hey, this isn't a thing you need to do alone . . . I know help can be a struggle to find and to afford but you deserve good care and you don't have to rawdog reality all by yourself." This is extra true when it comes to eating disorders. If only one thing has come across thus far in this book, I hope that it's how dangerous eating disorders are, how serious they are, and how complex they are to treat.

So this section includes some of the work I include in my practice around a brain that has been at war with its own body. And this is valuable eating disorder recovery work. We're going to start by talking about professional help you can get for eating disorders (and in case it wasn't clear the other eleventy billion times I said it, I strongly recommend professional help!). Then I'm going to give you a bunch of different exercises and interventions that I use in my practice in support of the management and recovery of disordered eating and disordered body image.

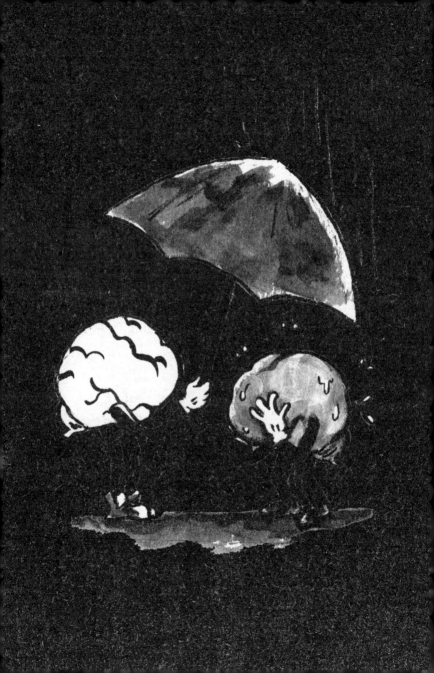

PROFESSIONAL TREATMENT

*E*ating disorders are so fucking hard to treat. This is not a newsflash, even within this book. It's important for me to keep restating this, however, because it's also so easy to feel hopeless in the face of such complexity. But you aren't a failure if you've struggling to access appropriate care and support for your healing journey. Eating disorder treatment is complex because the disease is, and there isn't going to be one singular mechanism of healing.

If you are struggling with food and body image, whether or not you think you meet the criteria for a full-blown eating disorder, seeking professional help is going to be a key part of your recovery.

Part of the overwhelm in this regard can be to whom you go for help. A specialist? Your primary care provider? A hotline? Your therapist? Where do you start? There's no correct answer except: With the person you trust most to believe you and follow through. They may not be a clinician at all, but a teacher or friend who you know can steer you in the right direction. Wherever you start, you're likely to end up seeing multiple professionals and using multiple strategies. But you're always going to need someone in your corner that knows *you*, not just the particular constellation of what you are struggling with.

Psychotherapy

Talk therapy is obviously the big one. Individual and group therapy have both been found to be effective in eating disorder treatment. Cognitive Behavioral Therapy (CBT) and Dialectical Behavioral Therapy (DBT) tend to be most commonly used because they focus on the interplay of thoughts and feelings and how they impact our behaviors. CBT is the gold standard treatment for body dysmorphic disorder because it focuses on creating a more balanced view of your own body. DBT adds more distress tolerance and mindfulness skills which are particularly helpful for some types of disordered eating.

Talk therapy externalizes our issues in a literal way. You've probably heard the expression "you're only as sick as your secrets." Part of that is because silence means we are living in a place of shame, with the belief that no one can be trusted to hear the messy parts and still love us. And that is awful enough. But also? All of these secret thoughts and feelings and sensations are a huge tangled ball of string when they sit up in there. I will tell my clients, "let's pick at the threads of this," which is our shorthand for "keep talking, I'll help you untangle." Someone with a new perspective can help you see patterns and timelines, and maybe provide new insight into motivations. They can help you figure out what best serves you and what does not. Therapy is a process of discernment . . . which isn't always just about what's right and what's wrong. It's also about teasing out what's right and what's almost right. Therapy helps you build skills, knowledge, and insight into the issues life has served forth so you have a better chance at being a happy, healthy human.

Your therapist should be someone you trust and feel comfortable with. If you request clarification on the questions they ask, they should be able to answer you. Like, "That is an exception-seeking question. I'm curious about times that you *did* feel that you handled a situation effectively so we can map over those skills to the area in which you are struggling."

Every therapist has a different style of working. The fancy term for this is "theoretical orientation," which only means "there is a plan behind the bullshit that comes out of my mouth."[13] I'm not super prescriptive on therapeutic

13 And for what it's worth? If there is no plan behind what comes out of your therapist's mouth? You absolutely need a new therapist. That's not

orientations and which ones work best for which issues. It provides a framework that a competent therapist uses to map their strategies. But that doesn't mean you can't have a kind of therapy that makes sense *for you*. Maybe you've read a lot about how dialectical behavior therapy or acceptance and commitment therapy is helpful and you resonate with that approach? Definitely look for a therapist that specializes in that and can communicate how they work clearly. The longer someone has been in the field, the more modalities they have likely trained in and can operate from, and can share their different ideas with you while you develop your treatment plan together.

Medical and Psychiatric Treatment

If someone has been struggling with disordered eating, especially for a longer period of time, medical care is going to be fundamental to mental health care because it is far easier for a healthy body to emotionally recover than a sick and starving one.

Your doctor is an important part of your recovery team. Because eating disorders have such direct and serious physical health consequences, there are likely to be some needed medical tests and treatments on top of the nutritional support the body needs to be functioning in

eclecticism, that's chaos.

good health again. For example, they may treat bone density loss caused by a long term nutritional deficit. Along with other trained clinicians, they can suggest supplementation to help stabilize needed minerals like iron and magnesium as well as helping mitigate inflammation. Other medical needs can include cardiac care, care for other harmed organs, and care for bone density loss.

Your doctor or psychiatrist can also prescribe medications in support of your recovery. One of the first considerations of prescription medications should be the treatment of any co-occurring disorders. Mood and anxiety disorders are the most common, and efficacious treatment is both important for its own sake and for the sake of more successful eating disorder treatment.

Psych meds are sometimes used in some specific eating disorder presentations, and can sometimes be effective outside their initial intended use. For example, antidepressants do assist in weight gain with people who need to regain their set point, as can some antipsychotics (olanzapine has been studied the most therefore is used more often). Because the side effects of antipsychotics are serious, they are typically only given with more severe cases of anorexia. And this is one of those places where making sure physical health is re-stabilized is super important . . . especially with anorexia, the body is so shut down that it can't absorb medications well at all, so refeeding is foundational to any other medications being effective.

There are a few more psych meds that can help support bulimia recovery. Fluoxetine, dosed at 60mg, has been shown to be incredibly effective at managing both the binge and purge cycles of bulimia. Other medications that have been found to be helpful with these behaviors include tricyclic antidepressants and monoamine oxidase inhibitors. Buspar, a non-sedative anxiety medication has also been shown to be effective. There haven't been as many studies of antipsychotics for bulimia treatment, though one involving lithium was found to be entirely ineffective.

For binge eating disorder, the anti-emetic medication ondansetron has been found to be helpful, but the most commonly used medication for BED is topiramate, which is actually an anticonvulsant. Topiramate tamps down hunger signals in many of the people who take it, so it makes it harder to binge and many people who have gained weight due to BED find that their bodies return to their normal set point, as well. The dosage range suggested by research is 25-600mg a day, which is a wildly variant number. But as someone who has taken this particular medication for migraines, I can testify that dosing is a PITA and will likely take a lot of adjustments, but is well worth the process if you start noticing some results.

For body dysmorphic disorder, serotonin uptake inhibitors are the best line of defense. This includes fluoxetine, escitalopram, fluvoxamine, sertraline, paroxetine, and clomipramine. These medications are typically dosed higher than they would be for major depression. Because of this, citalopram is not recommended, because the Federal Drug Administration (FDA) limits the dose to 40 mg a day (and half that if you are over age 60), and if you have BDD you typically need a higher dose than the FDA allowed maximum.

Nutritional Support

Working with a dietician or other licensed professional with specific nutrition training is invaluable for recovery. Not because *"we're going to explain why food and calories are important"* (we fuckin' know, thanks) but to help with everything that needs to happen around refeeding a starving body. A body that has been particularly nutritionally deprived for a length of time mostly needs nourishment, which is the first goal.

But refeeding often is incredibly uncomfortable at first, physically and emotionally. Physically, people often feel full and sick because their bodies aren't used to taking in appropriate caloric content.[14] Additionally, all of the

14 And oftentimes have to take in more than an average amount of food.

feelings that the disordered behavior was masking start coming to the surface because they can no longer be masked . . . causing more emotional distress.

Besides physical discomfort, refeeding can lead to what is known as refeeding syndrome, which also needs to be carefully monitored for by a professional treatment provider, especially in the first four days after someone starts eating and drinking again. When a starved body starts getting consistent food again, our blood sugar can go haywire, affecting our already low stores of phosphorus, potassium, magnesium, calcium, and sodium in the bloodstream and causing a serious electrolyte imbalance and a whole host of problems, potentially including organ failure.

The first signs of this condition are lightheadedness and fatigue (as well as blood pressure and heart rate dysregulation), making it really easy to miss if you're not being monitored for it. Which is, yes, me saying that professional support during this process is *really* important. Because I am a clinical nutritionist, I do have a BP cuff and stethoscope in my office, but still don't attempt refeeding

---

Refeeding can lead to a short term ramping up of the metabolism which means some people end up losing more weight in refeeding and need more calories just to maintain, let alone gain. All the research about why this happens hasn't found an answer. The book *Sick Enough* refers to this as the black box of eating disorder research because the mechanisms surrounding this response remain opaque.

with anyone who has been depleted for any measure of time. Treatment generally includes intravenous electrolytes, then continued electrolytes and vitamins until lab work shows stabilization.

That being said? Sometimes a client of mine hits a rough patch, and responds with a couple weeks of restricting as a means of control. When they come in for their next session and they tell me what's been going on, we will do some in-office refeeding along with the breathwork that helps food stay down (this technique is included later in the book, I'm not holding out on ya, promise).

Another thing a nutritionist can help you with is when you have to deal with very real dietary restrictions, whether for medical, religious, or moral reasons. For example one of the most common refeeding foods is chocolate milk. If you're allergic to dairy, that wouldn't be appropriate for you. So while intuitive eating type programs say "no food is off the table," sometimes it still is for a variety of reasons that have nothing to do with eating disorder restriction.

As a nutritionist, here are some of the things I try to do around dietary restrictions:

1) I ask frankly about any history of disordered eating and dieting. If a client has a history, I prefer other methods of treatment rather than a limited diet that will reactivate disordered eating. We

can work with supplementation or something else instead. Every once in a while someone with this history is struggling so much with other issues that we agree to try a food plan, but my monitoring of their emotional health and eating behaviors is far more stringent.

2) I reinforce that I am a "non-scale-victory" clinical nutritionist. Meaning, I'm not your girl for a weight loss plan. Our goals around nutrition will be alleviation of symptoms, more energy, more physical endurance, better lung capacity, whatever. We will not be discussing the numbers that show up on a scale when you stand on it as if that reinforces some kind of value about you and your body.

3) If you are hungry on any kind of plan, real cellular hunger, you need to fucking eat something. Refer back to the previous rule, we aren't looking at caloric restriction.

4) Any food plan is going to be built around what you like to eat. This blows people's minds when they ask me to help them set up a food plan and my response is "Sure! What do you like to eat?" rather than prescribing kale or whatever. We can

build a plan that includes more anti-inflammatory foods while letting you still have stuff you enjoy.

5) Strict limitation forever isn't the goal, healing is. There are some things I really can't eat at all but plenty of others I can now manage better as my body has healed over the years. We want to be looking at ways of introducing a wider variety of foods back into your diet sooner rather than later.

When working with a nutritionist, your eating and body history should be taken into account, and there should be flexibility and consideration for your likes, dislikes, and budget. Exercise should be joyful not punishing. And food should still be fucking delicious.

And what if weight loss really is necessary? Sometimes there is a direct line between weight and a particular medical issue. It's rare, but at times a doctor may order weight loss in preparation for an upcoming surgery, like some knee surgeries. Any weight loss should be slow and careful. **No starvation diets.** That's just prescribing to someone with a larger body what we treat in a smaller one. And, as established in neon lights, telling anyone to starve themselves is patently ridiculous.

Group Therapy and Programs

Groups can be incredibly helpful to recovery, whether a therapy group (something run by a clinician) or a peer-support group (a group that consists entirely of people with lived experience that runs itself). Group therapy is generally much cheaper than individual therapy, while most peer groups cost nothing, only requesting donations to help manage direct expenses for snacks, meeting rooms, etc. Being with others who can relate to both your story and your determination to heal can be instrumental to your own success, because you get understanding, support, and accountability.

In the Resources section at the end of this book, I've listed a number of eating disorder groups. You may notice that most of these are process/support groups that are sponsored by well-known eating disorder organizations. If you join one of these groups, you can expect that it will be run by a clinician. An open process group still gives you the flexibility to discuss anything you are working through, but within parameters of safety set by the group leader. Some groups are more structured and you may be working through a workbook together or something similar.

Another option that a lot of people consider are programs such as Overeaters Anonymous (OA), based on the 12-step abstinence model of Alcoholics Anonymous. There have been some rigorous studies of 12-step models for substance-related issues and they have consistently shown some efficacy is promoting both short and long term recovery and resilience. Many people ascribe the fellowship of other individuals with lived experience to be of great benefit to their sobriety. And these are the types of groups in which there is no cost to participate, making these often the most widely accessible option for support. But there are some pitfalls to be aware of.

As we have already established, it is doubtful that food is an addictive substance, even when it often feels that way from the inside. And this is likely why there is no rigorous evidence that these 12 step programs around food are equally helpful for disordered eating.

The real danger is when these groups start foisting food plans on members. Back in 1997, OA made a rule against groups endorsing or sharing specific food plans. But that hasn't stopped certain groups from defining what food addiction abstinence should look like, not just in terms of eating behaviors but what we are allowed to eat . . . rather than leaving that part of recovery to the participant and their professional support team. And, as we already discussed in great detail, the most efficacious approach to treating eating disorders is not based on the exclusion of huge categories of food.

This food-plan-foisting is thought to be even more common with other 12-step eating disorder programs like Anorexics and Bulimics Anonymous (ABA), Compulsive Eaters Anonymous (CEA), CEA-Honesty, Openness, Willingness (CEA-HOW), Eating Disorders Anonymous (EDA), and Food Addicts Anonymous (FAA). The concern is that when we impose a strict diet like this, we are teaching people to trade one kind of disordered eating for another. And it's foundationally at odds with current clinical guidelines.

So proceed with caution if you are investigating these options. My own mom was involved in OA for most of her adult life and found the support helpful for binge eating issues. But if people affiliated with the group try to shove you into an eating behavior that is at odds with the work you are doing with clinicians, either run like the wind or bring the plan back to the clinician in question and ask their advice

And this is true for *any* group that states they exist to support eating disorder recovery. There are wonderful groups and shady shit in equal numbers, so protect your emotional wellness and your peace by not getting roped into anything that goes against all the work you are trying to do.

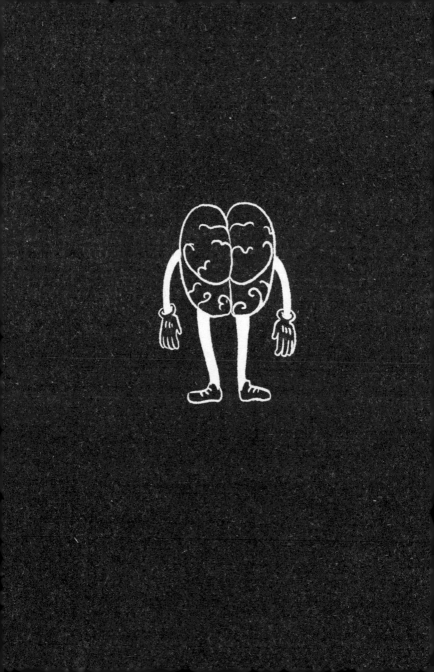

UNFUCKING OUR RELATIONSHIP WITH SELF

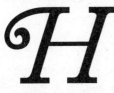opefully, I've convinced you that getting quality medical and clinical treatment is essential. But it isn't the end point of recovery. And I'm not going to try to convince you to love yourself if you feel so far removed from the possibility of doing so . . . I know how hard that is. But I hope you can make connections to how you think, feel, and perceive your body, which will help you start moving to a healthier relationship with it.

In this chapter, we're focusing on stuff you can do with your therapist, in a support group, or even on your own. There are exercises to help you zero in on how you talk to yourself, how you feel about yourself, and how the outside world influences both. Things that are simple, but not easy.

But it won't be any harder than living in a body that feels like the enemy without giving up on yourself. Which means, you're strong AF and you deserve to use that strength in support of thriving instead of surviving.

Softening the Critical Voice

Ok, let's be honest. It's just us here, after all, right?

How do you talk to yourself when you fuck up, or even think you might have fucked up or that you might fuck up in the future?

What kind of nasty things do you say? What tends to trigger that experience for you? How well do you connect to others after shitting all over yourself?

Kristen Neff, author of the book *Self-Compassion*, says, "If you are continually judging and criticizing yourself while trying to be kind to others, you are drawing artificial boundaries and distinctions that only lead to feelings of separation and isolation." That's a big thing there.

We are all trying to find that balance between caring for our bodies and making healthy choices without falling into a disordered behavior, right? Researchers studying self-compassion have demonstrated time and again that we take far better care of ourselves in the long run and are far more successful at our goals if we don't try to hate ourselves into submission.

In case you are wondering, self-compassion is very different from the concept of self-esteem. Self-esteem tells you to hype yourself up with praise that often feels temporary at best and empty at worst. Self-compassion is about recognizing your own humanity, connecting to the humanity of others, and loving your flawed self enough that you are worthy of respect, care, and nourishment.

Self-compassion work has been found to be especially efficacious in eating disorder recovery, especially with BED. We are just better connected to our own human experience and the world around us when we are compassionate with ourselves.

What kind of shift would you create in yourself if you treated yourself like your best friend instead of your worst enemy?

What if your best friend had fucked up hardcore? You would be compassionate, wouldn't you? You wouldn't let them off the hook, but you would help them take responsibility, try to fix the mess they made, and remind them that they are a human being, after all. And human beings fail. Now imagine if your best friend made a small mistake. Would you shame and punish them? Now imagine hearing your best friend heap shame and hatred on their own body. How would you want to hear them talking about themself?

Give yourself the same compassion you would give someone you love.

So, instead of:

"I can't believe that bullshit you pulled, why are you even on this planet??"

Try:

"Wow, OK, so that didn't work out. Everything went sideways. I need to figure out the best thing to do now to try to fix as much as possible. And figure out why it went sideways so I can try to avoid it happening again. I feel like shit right now, but I can learn from this and fail differently, and fail better, next time."

Instead of:

"You are gross AF, all you did was eat nachos and play Switch all weekend, no wonder you can't even catch a date."

Try:

"I'm really feeling unwell this morning. I'm lethargic and bloated and I don't enjoy being in my body like that. My food and movement choices weren't well balanced this weekend, but I can make a better choice starting today. I'm gonna skip the fries at lunch and hit the gym on my way home. Even if I just watch the news while walking the treadmill, I know it'll go a long way into feeling strong and having more energy."

Or, instead of:

> "Maybe if you stock up on protein shakes and creatine, then hire a trainer at the gym and go for two hours every morning, you can build enough muscle mass to not suck ass on the soccer field."

Try:

> "Is soccer important to me? Is it even fun? Do I enjoy it? Can I enjoy it without being perfect? What's a reasonable amount of effort to put into being better at something and amping my sense of accomplishment without losing my damn mind?"

The Abandoned Self

The three fundamental causes of human suffering have been described by physician William Shaver as isolation, loss of significance, and self-abandonment. Much of the work I do with individuals in eating disorder recovery is recognizing the connection between self-abandonment and disordered eating. *Abandonment* is the cessation of connection. It's a disengagement in the most complete sense of the word. Self-abandonment is the continuous mistrust and/or suppression of your own internal voice. It's coupled with a rejection of your own needs, desires, thoughts, feelings, and boundaries. But you are also vigilant about considering the needs, desires, thoughts, feelings, and boundaries of others.

Self-abandonment is a learned behavior that is often the result of childhood experiences of abuse, neglect, or invalidation. The development of a personal sense of self in childhood is critical to a healthy adulthood. If we receive the message that our internal world is not valued and important, we learn to put it aside. And if we can no longer relate to ourselves with care and consideration, we develop strategies to ease the pain of this disconnect. We don't feel safe in the world, and all of our processes and motivations stem from that place. Which then, leads to more detachment (being aloof and disinterested), dysregulation (being out of control of your physical and emotional self), dissociation (feeling disconnected from your own body), and intense suffering (continued distress).

What does self-abandonment feel like internally?

- Mistrusting your instincts. Maybe you let others make decisions for you even though they don't know more than you do about the situation. Or you might catch yourself perseverating and second-guessing both your sense of self and your choices

- People pleasing by centering others at the expense of your own needs, wants, and desires

- Hiding or diminishing aspects of yourself, including your feelings, interests, beliefs, hopes, and dreams

- Having unrealistic expectations of what you should be able to accomplish, while still never feeling you have done enough even when you succeed at these goals

- Feeling critical and judgmental about yourself instead of kind and caring

- Suppressing your feelings because you are afraid they will be considered wrong or that you'll be judged harshly for them

- Acting out of alignment with your own values

When we live in a state of constant hypervigilance and dysregulation, we look for compensatory means of creating a sense of safety in our lives. This may take one of the following forms:

- Seeking of money, power, or fame

- Feeling unstable without a relationship that you use in place of self-regulation.

- Engaging in short-term energy relieving behaviors (STERBS) to cope with the internal experiencing of dysregulation (such as substance use disorders, eating disorders, or out-of-control behaviors around things like shopping, sex, or internet usage)

When we talk about self-abandonment, I refer to this state as the "protected self." There is nothing wrong with protecting yourself, and when you took on this it was the only way you *could* protect yourself. But over time, the cost gets higher and higher. Self-protection means ignoring your own wants, needs, and desires in the interest of placating others. Over time, you stop remembering what those wants, needs, and desires actually even are. The opposite of this state is a healed, integrated self, where you have space to be honest about your life, both your struggles and your victories, because you can trust your fundamental goodness.

Knowing the research around how self-abandonment presents led me to create a model that breaks down the components of both a protected, abandoned self and a healed, integrated self so I could better guide my clients through their healing work.

This is all based on practice-based evidence, not evidence-based practice. Meaning, there is no research behind this model (as of yet). It is created based on the experiences I have had as a therapist. It may be helpful in guiding your own work or you may say, "meh, doesn't suit" and move on.

Components of a Protected Self

Emotionally Dysregulated: Emotional dysregulation occurs when we have little or no capacity to cope with painful or uncomfortable emotions. Because an abandoned self is not allowed the full range of emotional experiences, as these emotions may be ridiculed or denied by others and feel uncomfortable to express an ownership of.

Self-Loathing: Self-loathing, simply put, is a core hatred of oneself. It may not always present in the form of low self-worth; it can also look like a huge surface ego that has been propped into place to hide the truth of our relationship to self.

Morally Indeterminate: This means we de-center our own moral code in service of pleasing others. It occurs when our own behaviors are not in line with what we consider to be valuable and important to the world.

Relicf-Seeking: Relief seeking behaviors are anything that gives us a little biochemical hit of happiness or calm when we feel not much of either. As mentioned above, this often takes the form of short-term energy relieving behaviors (STERBS) which allow us to discharge some of the frustrations of not living authentically and fully.

Performative: Performative behaviors are those that we take solely with our audience in mind, to elicit a certain response from them. Meaning, we act the way we want others to see rather than from a place of what we truly value.

Components of an Integrated Self

Emotionally Conscious: An emotionally conscious person is aware of their responses and allows themselves to feel and work through their feelings, even ones that are painful and uncomfortable.

Self-Compassionate: A self compassionate person accepts themself with all the complexities of the human experience. They don't let themself off the hook for making ungreat choices, but recognize them as a learning process that we must go through in order to continue to work toward being the best humans we possibly can.

Morally Aligned: A morally aligned person has a strong sense of right and wrong and operates from these principles even in the face of disagreement from others.

Purpose Directed: A purpose directed person has a clear idea of what they contribute to the world and their own joy in living. They function from this place rather than one of fear and self-criticism, even when doing so is difficult.

Authentic: An authentic person speaks from their own truth, with kindness and ownership, rather than performing the role that others expect from them.

Reconnection to Self

If you're reading the protected self model above and thinking, "check, check, check," that may seem liked a pretty fucked situation from which it seems impossible to break free. Identifying a protected self is a large part of therapeutic work, but with a goal of healing, not beating yourself up about it.

Healing is absolutely possible—for everyone. Awareness of what we are working toward is the majority of the battle. And giving ourselves space and validation to reclaim ourselves is the rest of it. We need space to be validated in our pain. Hidden pain shatters, but seen pain heals. When someone is able to hold space for our messiness, that shows us that imperfection doesn't make us unloveable and doesn't need to be corrected to a behavior that is smaller and more palatable to others. It says (as does the art on the wall in my office), *"You belong here and everything you feel is alright."*

We can absolutely hold that space for ourselves, but it's deeply powerful coming from another person—even if that isn't necessarily the person you hoped it would be. This is part of the reason that healing works much better in community than alone and why I encourage anyone going through this process to find a support group that focuses on these underlying issues to join if you can't afford individual therapy.

The pragmatic part of reintegrating a hidden self requires a lot of slowing down, checking in with oneself, and becoming more radically self-honest. It requires thinking through our responses to people and situations so we can change our unthinking earlier patterns. It means building up an arsenal of new responses and using them, even when it is uncomfortable to do so, over and over again, until it becomes our new normal.

For example, when faced with a task, decision, or expectation, what happens when you ask yourself:

1) What necessitates this decision? Are uncomfortable emotions pushing me to think I need to do or be something? Do I really need to act, or do I need to slow down and feel?

2) If I had an "easy button" to get myself out of this situation, would I use it? If I could say "no" without hurting someone's feelings or causing issues, would I do so without hesitation? What would happen if I just took a deep breath and said no?

This is a difficult skill at first. And at second, third, and fourth. That's ok. When we have *years* of practice relating to the world one way, it takes time to build new neural pathways. You're not a failure if you have to work on this. Keep going—you can choose low-stakes situations to practice, or even role-play with friends. The more success you are able to build up, the more efficacious you will feel about the process.

Questions for consideration

- Did anything within these models resonate with you as being an accurate depiction of your experiences with self-abandonment?

- Did anything seem inaccurate? What would be more spot-on for you?

- Where might there be some opportunity to reconnect to your authentic self?

- What might you gain in the process?

Social Media Detox Week

So you know how we talked about the way exposure to media depictions of really thin people is a high risk factor for eating disorders? Spending a lot of time on social media can really get into your head the same way. That shit can be toxic to your self-image because you're constantly comparing yourself to others, even subconsciously . . . and all that scrolling makes it hard to tune into your body. I'm not going to ask you to firebomb your accounts, or even take an entire day off social media—so many of us rely on it for our work, friendships, and community. But give yourself a week to change the way you engage with it and see how you feel.

Day One: Pay attention to the number of times you pick up/open up/use your phone, tablet, laptop, etc. during the day.

Day Two: Yesterday's number? Cut that in half. THE PAINNNNNNN!

Day Three: Eat all meals and snacks mindfully, instead of scrolling on your phone, tablet, laptop while eating.

Day Four: No phone for the first 45 minutes after waking up.

Day Five: No social media scrolling for two hours before bedtime.

Day Six: Call someone you usually only connect with on social media or by text. Scary, I knooooow! But hey, maybe even just leave them a message like "I saw the picture from your fishing trip and realized we haven't chatted in forever, and I would love to catch up!"

Day Seven: Reflect. What is your relationship with your own body today? Is anything different just from making some small detox changes? Anything you want to make a habit?

Body Neutrality

Our relationships with our own bodies are a huge part of our emotional wellness. And there is so much media discussion around body positivity. But that is often a very high bar that takes a long time to learn how to clear. So I teach my clients (and remind myself) to aim for *body neutrality*. You don't have to embrace and adore every aspect of your body in order to appreciate how hard it works to keep you going despite every obstacle you have faced.

This activity is designed to help you build upon your sense of embodiment and enhance your comfort and acceptance of your external, physical presentation of self.

This activity is adapted from my book *Unfuck Your Intimacy*, because (unshockingly) body image is also a huge issue in our intimate relationships. You can do it all by yourself or with a trusted partner, friend, or therapist.

If you are working with a partner, discuss in advance their role in the process. The important thing is that they listen to you rather than correct your thoughts and feelings about your body. We often want to tell people we care about how we perceive them, and we often see them with much less criticism than they see themselves. It's hard not to say something akin to "No! I love your neck!"

But the point of the exercise is to share our own internal experience without fear of argument or correction.

It is also not your partner's job to ask questions or give feedback about your experience. The partner's job is to provide a supportive presence. If appropriate, they can then complete the activity with your support as well. It's amazing what you will learn about each other, if you are in a place where you feel safe enough to do this activity together.

Stand in front of a full-length mirror, wearing whatever clothing feels comfortable (as much or as little as you'd like). Take a deep breath and look at your body in its entirety for a few minutes. If this isn't something you often do, give yourself time to become accustomed to the experience.

Next, starting at the top of your head and moving downward, describe each part of your body and the feelings you have about it. Say everything you are thinking out loud, even if you're doing this activity alone. It is amazing how much we say to ourselves that we are not very aware of, because we don't give literal voice to those thoughts and feelings.

When you're done, ask yourself some of these questions:

- What did you notice about yourself? Did anything you notice surprise you? Did anything you found yourself saying out loud surprise you?

- If you were to pick out one or two body parts or areas that you most dislike, what would these be and why?

- If you were to pick out one or two body parts or areas that are your favorite, what would they be and why?

- Did your perceptions of yourself shift when you moved from looking at your entire body to focusing on parts of it at a time? If so, in what ways?

- If you did this activity with a partner, you can ask your partner to answer the following questions: What surprised them about your experience? Did you say anything they didn't expect? Did they notice that you ignored any areas? Did you express any thoughts or feelings that they weren't aware of?

More body neutrality tips:

- Focus on an aspect of yourself that is separate from the destructive body image messages you are combating. For instance, if you're hypercritical of your physical self, try focusing on your strong self, playful self, or sensual self. Consider these a different dimension from what you are unhappy about.

- Focus on your body in its entirety, rather than certain parts. Look at yourself (and if you're doing this with a partner, ask them to look at you) with "soft eyes," or focusing on the entirety of what is wonderful about you. This may be easier to hold onto as truth, instead of pulling out positive feelings about specific aspects of your body.

- Hold space for the possibility that even if you do not accept and love your body right now (or even struggle to feel neutral about it), it is possible to feel differently in the future. *"Not right now"* has far less a pervasive hold on us than *"never"* and allows small shifts to occur that move us in a healthy direction.

- Apologize (as authentically as possible, even if it feels cheesy) to your body for treating it like the enemy. For treating it like it is somehow a separate entity from the rest of you. Tell it you will work on incorporating it back into the whole and appreciate all it has done to keep you moving forward despite your negativity toward it.

UNFUCKING OUR RELATIONSHIP WITH FOOD

*E*verything above is about befriending your own body. And that's so incredibly important. But we also have to work with our bodies and the food they need to stay healthy and well. For those of us with an eating disorder history, that seems untenable to attempt and impossible to achieve. But it's vital work, and in this chapter we are going to get super practical about it.

We're going to delve deep into how to tell the difference between real hunger and emotional eating triggers. I'm going to give you some practical exercises for getting food down and keeping it down. We're going to get into mindful eating, not just breaking eating down into its simplest mechanical parts, but also something we can enjoy and take pleasure in again. And we're also going to talk about how to handle relapses, which are an incredibly common part of recovery.

Cellular Versus Emotional Hunger

One of the first things we lose in disordered eating is an ability to know our own bodies and what they need. Being able to tell the difference between true hunger and using food to soothe becomes increasingly difficult, especially

Emotional Hunger	Cellular Hunger
Sudden	Gradual
Specific food	Open to different foods
Urgent or overwhelming	Uncomfortable and needs to be addressed, but you can wait
Connected to an uncomfortable emotional state	Connected to a physical need for energy input
More automatic or mindless	More aware and mindful
Eats to (and past) the point of discomfort	Stops when satiated
Feels guilt, shame, and other negative emotions after eating	Feels positive, or at least neutral

when we are engaging in binging or mindless eating behaviors.

As someone who spent many years struggling to understand those two types of hunger, it was incredibly helpful for me to get very granular about their differences. Now I am in a place where I can sense the difference relatively simply. It was a hard road to walk but my relationship with food has shifted into an experience of it being a source of both fuel and pleasure rather than a mechanism for stuffing discomfort.

In this model, cellular hunger refers to the messages sent by a body that needs energy to maintain stasis, and emotional hunger is a craving to eat as a way to distract from or manage our own internal processes.

When you look at this list, what habits did you realize you can relate to? How can you build more presence around these habits as you start to untangle emotional hunger from cellular hunger?

The 5 Emotional Hungers

Let's talk about emotional hunger more—because it's such a big issue at the core of so much disordered eating, and there is far more than just one motivation, feeling, or reason behind it.

Emotional eating is a behavior in which we eat past our physiological need for sustenance, often choosing foods with a palatable and soothing mouth-feel which are energy-dense (read: higher in quick energy calories). It may be undertaken as a direct means of coping with negative emotions, or because the emotions themselves have created a strong physiological response in the body that is mistaken for hunger.

The almost universal experience of emotional eating has very little academic research behind it despite it being a common theme in all of our media. The unhappy girl taking out a pint of ice cream after a crappy day at work. Or the entire pizza and bag of cookies after a bad breakup. We can all nod in recognition but if you look for empirical data . . . there isn't much. And what does exist focuses generally on people who have been labeled obese by BMI standards. The research on people of all shapes and sizes is scant. As is the research on people of all genders. And while depression is a factor that is often studied with emotional overeating, the other complexities of human existence are rarely mentioned.

While researching this book, I began to develop a theory that there are core emotional hungers that as humans we experience time and again. And if we could recognize them in our own lives we will have had a far better chance of nourishing ourselves in a different way.

When you look closely at the research on emotional eating that does exist, you see references not only to depression and anxiety, but also loneliness, boredom, stress, and worries. It's also related to a construct called "tense-tiredness," which I consider a level of overwhelm with which there is no hope for rest. Another big one was "confused mood" . . . meaning, "I feel unsettled but I don't even know how or why." And interestingly, a confused mood was expressed often by the boys and men who participated in research around this topic. The mechanisms by which we don't allow masculine individuals to experience and express a variety of uncomfortable emotions (remember hegemonic masculinity from earlier in the book?) has led to a literal confusion about what they are feeling, resulting in reaching desperately for anything that soothes that feeling.

So emotional eating is not just driven by depression. It's not just a function of "fatness" (however the fuck that is being defined this week by the powers that be). It's a common human experience. Food is generally readily available and plentiful, at least in industrialized places. It becomes the cheapest and easiest means of feeling better when we feel awful.

And then the greatest irony is that when we emotionally overeat, we cease to enjoy what we eat. It is providing a sense of relief, but it really isn't delicious. Or nourishing. Or something we share with those we love. We lose out on the human joy of being alive and present in our body while providing it with energy and care.

Reclaiming that experience starts with recognizing the difference between emotional hunger and physical hunger. Then working to provide ourselves the nourishment we are really craving. Since that can feel like a very overwhelming prospect, this model is designed to offer a language and a structure to better recognize how our own lives are being impacted by all of our non-physical hungers. If you're interested in working through this concept more in-depth, I have a workbook zine called *The Five Emotional Hungers*. For purposes of this book, here's what we're looking for:

Hunger for Relief: *A release from anxiety or distress. A reassurance of survival.* For example, if your partner says, "We need to talk when I get home," and you still have a few hours until they actually come home, and your mind is spinning disasters, eating the entire box of Girl Scout cookies may suddenly seem like a really good idea.

Hunger for Equanimity: *A mental calmness. A brain break in the midst of chaos. A moment to regain composure. A sense of peaceful acceptance of what is, good or bad.* For example, work has been nonstop and exhausting for hours, you haven't had time to stop and think or even take a deep breath. And then, *holy shit*, there is a bag of hot cheetos calling your name right now.

Hunger for Control: *A re-empowerment. The ability to make decisions for oneself instead of being narrated by others.* For example, you just got blessed out by your family for something that happened years ago. But there is no telling your auntie to back the fuck off for once. And she did bring her famous mashed potatoes loaded with cream cheese.

Hunger for Connection: *A need to be seen, heard, held, and understood. A desire for companionship and a shared experience.* For example, you've been in some level of pandemic quarantine for what seems like an endless amount of time. Or you are at school, away from all the people who have known you your whole life. You may be alone or not, but def lonely. And there doesn't seem to be any way to feel better at 2am than cold pizza and Netflix.

Hunger for Meaning: *A desire for purpose in the world. The ability to impact those around us for the better.* For example, you've been stuck in a job for some time that seems endless. It doesn't align with your goals, values, and what you want to do in the world. All of a sudden, that stale Thai takeout from last week that is sketch and should be thrown out looks delicious.

If you're a human being on planet Earth, you have likely experienced at least one (if not all) of these hungers. And they are clues to reconnecting to our hidden needs that have remained unmet. They help us see how we have devalued our own worth and the harmful ways we talk to ourselves about ourselves.

The way to work with these hungers is to create a sense of emotional safety that comes from within. You'll need to unpack them and try to figure out what's going on. Every time you tell yourself a harmful story about yourself or your behavior, imagine what the most loving person you can picture would tell you instead. It's okay if you don't quite believe it yet, you just need to create a space where it *might* be true. As you practice, return to the original hunger you were investigating. Has anything about it changed?

This can take a while and you might run into some dead ends. Emotional work is always a process, and never finished.

Questions for consideration

- How have these hungers shown up in your life?
- How have you tried to satisfy these hungers in the past?
- What have you done to try to satisfy them, whether by eating or other actions?
- What would be a loving and healthy alternative response that you could try?

Befriending Your Body with a Five Senses Meditation

This is a mindfulness practice designed to help ground you in the present moment through a deeper experience of your own body. This practice can help you feel more connected with your body and better able to recognize your authentic, cellular hungers, as well as moments of emotional distress. So let's start with thinking about experiences you find enjoyable that are related to each of your senses.

1) What do I enjoy the sight of?

2) The sound of?

3) The smell of?

4) The taste of?

5) What do I enjoy the feel of on my skin?

Now, center yourself in your present surroundings and pay attention to the input you are currently getting through these senses. What are you noticing that is enjoyable? What is neutral? What is undesirable?

What about this exercise was easiest for you? What was more of a struggle? What did you notice about yourself in the process?

Letting Ourselves Have Pleasure

I read a beautiful essay by Nigella Lawson recently. It was in response to the trolling she got for posting a picture of her lunch, a sesame broccoli and shrimp dish. I think that sounds fucking delicious, but of course the internet had opinions. She got multiple messages from people asking her why she was being "good" when she could have cake instead.

Nigella, who adores cake, didn't want cake for lunch. She wrote eloquently about how she is hugely invested in the joy of food . . . to the point that when looking at a menu, she literally imagines eating each item to gauge the pleasure she would get out of it before making a decision. And for that lunch, the sesame broccoli and shrimp was what she wanted.

Pleasure is an enormously important part of nourishing our bodies. Food is delicious. It can build community, connection, and joy. It isn't just fuel for our bodies and you shouldn't be pushed into thinking of it that way. And eating for pleasure does not have to mean eating things that society has labeled unhealthy, indulgent, or guilt-inducing. Eating cake can be a legitimate pleasure, and so can eating beautifully prepared vegetables (maybe even with some sesame oil and shrimp). The pleasure is all in understanding your body's hungers and how to feed them in a way that's authentic to you.

Some of the most deeply pleasurable experiences of eating can be had when eating with mindfulness and intent. This technique, which I've adapted from the Mindfulness Based Stress Reduction curriculum, is designed to create presence in consumption. In the training, they use a raisin. I suggest starting with a small piece of a type of food that you don't have strong feelings about to practice the intent. Then start trying it with foods that bring you pleasure so you can practice being in the experiential moment of enjoying eating.

- Place a few raisins in your hand. And no, you don't have to use raisins, any food will do. I've found that even people who don't like raisins are not bothered by them in this exercise. But if they really gross you out, grab something else.

- Pretend this is your first day on the planet. This is a new food that you have never seen before, and you are an alien explorer that is going to make scientific study of raisins and raisin-ness. Use all five of your senses to explore it. Turn it around with your fingers, notice the color, the tactile sensations. How does it fold or reflect light? What does it smell like when you hold it up to your nose? Does it make any sound if you apply pressure?

- You will start having thoughts of the "Why am I doing this? This is fucking weird" variety. Totally normal. Just recognize them as a thought you are having and bring yourself back to the activity.

- Bring the object slowly to your mouth. Notice how automatic it is for your hand to bring nourishment up to your mouth. Notice whatever anticipation you are experiencing. Is your mouth watering? Gently place the raisin on your tongue without biting down. Explore the sensation of the raisin in your mouth.

- When you are ready, bite down. Notice the taste that is released when doing so. Notice how you habitually move it to one side of your mouth over another. Slowly chew the raisin. Notice how it changes in texture, and flavor as you chew. When you feel ready to swallow, notice your conscious intention to do so. Pay attention to the sensation of it moving down your throat, to your esophagus.

How did the experience of eating differ when you did so mindfully? What did you notice? What did you enjoy? What was uncomfortable?

Strategies for Stuffing

I had a client who referred to compulsive overeating patterns as "stuffing," because she was aware that she was using food to stuff negative emotions back down rather than examine and contend with them. As someone else with a stuffing history, the term resonated and I've used it for over a decade now.

What you're doing may not be stuffing, however. We also have a tendency to eat when we are just . . . bored. It becomes a mindless behavior. When everyone's daily routine changed in one way or another in 2020 due to COVID, the amount of bored-wandery-snacky behavior became a common theme. Jenny Lawson, The Bloggess, referred to that hungry-bored overlap as "hored."

Either way, whether you're stuffing or hored, you aren't eating with intention. You are not choosing foods that are nourishing your body, soul, and relationships. You're eating stuff that makes you feel sluggish or sick later. And that's what you're looking to change.

Record what you eat for a week. Just jot down the time of day, what you ate, what was going on at the time, and the emotions you were experiencing. No need to do portions or calorie counts, that's not the point. But you can differentiate that, for example, if you grabbed a handful of crackers to take into the bedroom versus demolishing the entire box of them while sitting on the floor in your underwear.

Now ask yourself the following questions:

- Did you notice any predominant emotional states that seemed to lead to emotional eating or making un-mindful food choices?

- What about mindless/bored states? Hored eating?

- Any particular days or times of day (or night) that seem to be particularly activating for you?

- Any particular place?

- Any particular activity (like watching TV or visiting a relative you can't stand)?

- Any other external cues (like someone cooking, the sound of someone opening a bag of chips, or seeing a display of candy at the store)?

- Are certain foods being available a point of activation?

Once you know what activates the behavior you are trying to diminish, you can plan around it. For example, I don't keep big tubs of ice cream in the house. I am not anti-ice cream, but I want it to be a treat that I go out for and savor with portion control that my brain isn't capable of at home.

Here are some more ideas. And when I say ideas, I mean shit I need to do way better and maybe you do too.

1. Eat slowly. Take a bite, and put your utensil down on the plate while you focus on and savor that bite.

2. If possible, designate the place you sit and eat your meals. You may not have a table and chair in

a dining room available, but choose somewhere to be the "eating place." In my office I eat sitting at my desk but not in my therapist chair, which would connect sitting there to snacking, meaning I could easily start snacking all day.

3. Don't engage in other activities while you're eating. No watching TV, reading, scrolling, driving, etc. It's easy to lose track of how much you are eating and stop noticing your innate full signals. When you're distracted, you don't enjoy your food in the same way. You're also making a psychological connection between that activity and eating.

4. Use plates and bowls that properly represent your portion size. It helps keep your brain from saying "that's a crap amount of pie, it's only covering ⅓ of the plate, get more!"

5. Consider putting away the part of the food that's for later after you portion out your amount for your immediate meal. You can put it away in the fridge if you're at home or ask for a take-out container from the get-go at a restaurant. This adds a couple more steps to going for seconds, allowing you to think about whether you are still genuinely hungry or if you are acting out of habit.

6. Keep the treat choices tucked away, and the nutrient-dense good energy choices readily available. Use see-through containers or pretty bowls for things like fresh fruit in the fridge. If you know you are more likely to snack on something that is ready to go, prep healthy snacks (like carrot sticks or apple slices) and have them where your eyes will hit first (this is a mom trick AF).

7. Don't have a candy or snack bowl out where it is easy to graze from, or at least stock it with things you are less likely to binge on. The candy bowl in my office is full of lollipops. I can't take out a handful of them, so even if I grab one it's NBD. Reeses cups, on the other hand, would be a huge problem.

8. Pack healthy snacks for yourself so you are less likely to hit the drive-through or snack machine. It also is nice to have a good option readily available if you are hangry and low-bloodsugary. I keep snacks in my office and car for just such occasions.

9. Look at ways to change your routine. If you tend to head straight for the fridge after you get home from work, for example, try getting something to

drink, go through the mail, etc. for 20 minutes first instead.

10. Keep water with you whenever possible. So often we think we are hungry and we are legit just thirsty.

11. Give yourself 10-15 minutes to see if you are actually hungry or having an emotional craving. If it's a stuffing or hored craving, it will decrease as the minutes pass. This pause is helpful before eating more at meal time, as well. It takes a while for our brain to get the signal that the stomach is full which is why it's so easy to go from "still hungry" to "completely stuffed and feeling kinda sick." Giving your brain a chance to catch up can prevent feeling overstuffed.

12. I love the Michael Pollan manifesto "If you aren't hungry for an apple, you aren't really hungry." I use this a lot when I'm so sure I'm hungry for toast and jam. I ask myself if an apple would suffice and if the answer is no, that's a good indicator that I'm wanting to carb-stuff away some uncomfortable feelings.

13. If you are in a situation where it's really hard to avoid food triggers (me and buffets and holiday parties) you can use gymnema, an herb with an

acid component that blocks our sweet sensors. A lot of people take gymnema to help manage their blood sugar, but you can also roll a tablet around in your mouth to turn down the sweet sensors on your tongue and lessen your impulse to go into cookie monster mode.

Breathing to Prevent Upchuck

Because so many eating disorders include regurgitation (rumination disorder, bulimia, sometimes anorexia and ARFID), strategies to help calm that regurgitation response are invaluable. As anyone who has struggled with an eating disorder can tell you, the vomiting becomes preconscious over time. And keeping food down becomes something for which we have to have an intentional strategy.

The most commonly prescribed technique is diaphragmatic (belly) breathing. The diaphragm is a rounded-top muscle that sits at the base of the lungs. When we throw up, the diagram contracts. Diaphragmatic breathing helps it remain relaxed.

If you are struggling to keep food down, try laying on your back on a flat surface with your head supported and your knees slightly bent.

No worries if you can't do that right now, it totally works anyway. If you're in the middle of a coffee shop, you probably have to stay seated so as not to be weird AF.

Whether you're seated or lying down, place one of your hands on your upper chest and the other below your rib cage. This will help you feel your diaphragm move as you breathe.

Breathe out slowly through your mouth, which you should feel your stomach muscles under the hand you placed on your stomach.

Then lightly tighten those same stomach muscles, and let them drop down as you breathe out through your pursed lips. Your hand on your chest should remain as still as possible so you can tell you are working from your diaphragm, not your chest.

If regurgitation is something you have struggled with, try practicing this technique for several minutes several times a day. Like 5-10 minutes 3-4 a day if you want a specific number. Practice it when you are *not* eating until it becomes second nature so you can easily use it when you are eating to help the food stay down.

Relapse Prevention Plan

As I've said only eleventy billion times throughout this book, eating disorders are incredibly hard to treat and recover from. It isn't like a broken arm that, once healed, will quite likely stay healed unless you fall off the trampoline again.

Eating disorders are adaptations created to give us a sense of control over a life that feels out of control. So really careful management of your day to day life will be invaluable. Relapse happens to the best of us. It doesn't make you a failure, it makes you a human being who is still learning. So having a plan to prevent but also bounce back afterwards is so important so that you don't shame spiral down into oblivion every time you slip.

This relapse prevention plan will be entirely unique to you. Meaning you can fill out your signs that you're on track, your signs that you're getting into more dangerous territory, and early signs of relapse that signal you need help.

Grab a notebook or piece of paper, or open a document file—something you'll be able to easily find and look at regularly. And start planning.

- What are signs that you're on track? (*Examples: Enjoying a meal out without checking calorie counts online, having energy to focus on things I love*)

- What specific actions help you stay on track? (*Examples: Keeping healthy food on hand, making a granular self-care plan*)

- What signs alert you that you might be getting off track? (*Examples: Spending more time with obsessive thoughts about food, feeling unhappy with my body, limiting social interactions involving food*)

- What are your recovery strategies to manage higher-risk behavior? (*Examples: Making a therapy appointment, planning full, nutritive meals and eating them, limiting calorie-burning exercise*)

- What are signs that you're starting to relapse? (*Examples: Deciding to purge because I feel overfull, deciding to try a new, restrictive diet plan*)

- Which recovery strategies help you manage high-risk behavior? (*Examples: Look for a higher level of care, like an intensive outpatient program, access care for lost nutrients*)

- Who on your treatment team do you contact if your relapse was particularly severe?

CONCLUSION

*I*f you read this book to help yourself get a better handle on your eating and body image, good for you! I know I've said a lot about how hard this is, but also know that there is a path for recovery for you. It may not look like mine, and it doesn't need to.

If you read this book because you wanted to find help for someone else in your life who is struggling, I hope you came away from it, if nothing else, with a stronger sense of how eating and body image play out in your own life, and what you can do about that. I've written a lot about addiction and out of control behaviors, and like those and many other mental health issues, the very first and best thing we can do for the people around us is attend to our own health and wholeness.

Most of us struggle with disordered eating, eating disorders, and body image problems, whether that's a lowkey every day self-berating or a full-blown, medically dangerous eating disorder or body dysmorphia.

We can't control the fucked up aspects of the environment we live in, but we can find healing, emotional safety, and a powerful, embodied sense of self. We can examine our own fatphobia and what it means for ourselves, the people around us, and our culture at large. This might be the work of a lifetime. But doing it may save lives—our own and those who see us doing the work and take strength and inspiration from it.

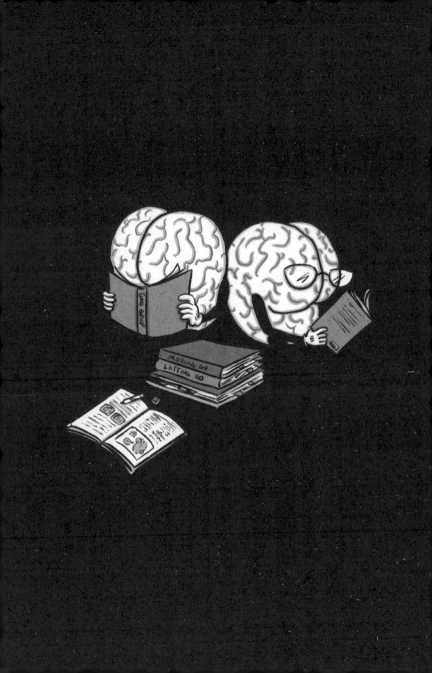

RESOURCES FOR SUPPORT

Eating Disorder Hotlines

Eating Disorders Awareness and Prevention (EDAP)

For answers to your questions, information, and nationwide referrals

Call or text 1-800-931-2237

Chat: nationaleatingdisorders.org

National Eating Disorder Referral and Information Center

edreferral.com

National Association of Anorexia Nervosa and Associated Disorders (ANAD)

Referrals to treatment, information, and support groups

(888)-375-7767 (Monday-Friday, 9:00am-9:00pm CST)

anad.org

The Renfrew Center

1-800-RENFREW (1-800-736-3739)

renfrewcenter.com

Free and Low Cost Eating Disorder Support

National Eating Disorders Association (NEDA) forums

nationaleatingdisorders.org/forum

NEDA Network virtual support groups

nationaleatingdisorders.org/neda-network-virtual-support-groups

ANAD (National Association of Anorexia Nervosa and Associated Disorders) support groups

anad.org/get-help/about-our-support-groups/

ANAD recovery mentors

anad.org/get-help/request-a-recovery-mentor/

The Alliance for Eating Disorders Awareness virtual support groups

allianceforeatingdisorders.com/

Maintenance Phase podcast

maintenancephase.com/

More Eating Disorder Resources

The Alliance for Eating Disorders

allianceforeatingdisorders.com/portal/home

Body Dysmorphic Disorder Foundation

bddfoundation.org/

National Association for Men With Eating Disorders

namedinc.org/

Trans Folx Fighting Eating Disorders (T-FEED)

transfolxfightingeds.org/

RECOMMENDED READING

Books about Dismantling Fatphobia

Body Respect: What Conventional Health Books Get Wrong, Leave Out, and Just Plain Fail to Understand about Weight by Lindo Bacon and Lucy Aphramor

The Obesity Myth: Why America's Obsession with Weight is Hazardous to Your Health by Paul Campos

What We Don't Talk About When We Talk About Fat by Aubrey Gordan

The Belly of the Beast: The Politics of Anti-Fatness as Anti-Blackness by Da'Shaun L. Harrison

Fat Politics: The Real Story behind America's Obesity Epidemic by J. Eric Oliver

Fearing the Black Body: The Racial Origins of Fat Phobia by Sabrina Strings

Books about Healing

Radical Belonging: How to Survive and Thrive in an Unjust World (While Transforming it for the Better) by Lindo Bacon

Embodiment and the Treatment of Eating Disorders: The Body as a Resource in Recovery by Catherine Cook-Cottone

Sick Enough: A Guide to the Medical Complications of Eating Disorders by Jennifer L. Gaudiani

Unfuck Your Body: Using Science to Eat, Sleep, Breathe, Move, and Feel Better by Faith G. Harper

Gentle Nutrition: A Non-Diet Approach to Healthy Eating by Rachael Hartley

Eating in the Light of the Moon: How Women Can Transform Their Relationship with Food through Myths, Metaphors, and Storytelling by Anita Johnston

Detox Your Masculinity: How Cultural Bullshit Fucks Up Men's Body Image (zine) by Aaron Sapp and Faith G. Harper

Self-Compassion: The Proven Power of Being Kind to Yourself by Kristen Neff

Body Kindness: Transform Your Health from the Inside Out and Never Say Diet Again by Rebecca Scritchfield

Your Body Is Not an Apology: The Power of Radical Self-Love by Sonja Renee Taylor

Your Body Is Not an Apology Workbook: Tools for Living Radical Self-Love by Sonja Renee Taylor

Intuitive Eating: A Revolutionary Program that Works by Evelyn Tribole and Elyse Resch

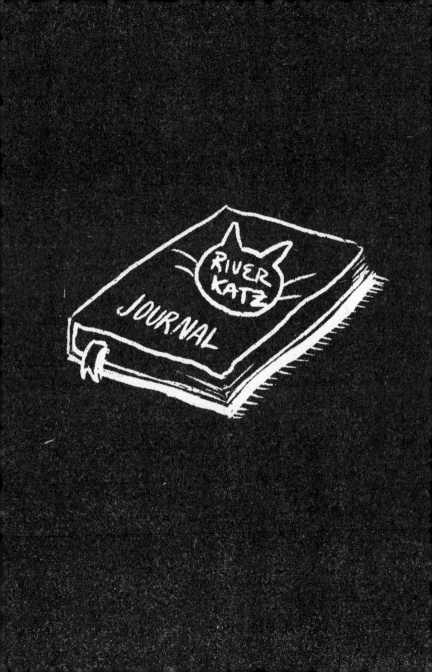

Citations

10 principles of intuitive eating. Intuitive Eating. (2019, December 19). Retrieved August 3, 2022, from intuitiveeating.org/10-principles-of-intuitive-eating/ Aeonmag. (n.d.). Blaming individuals for obesity may be altogether wrong: Aeon essays. Aeon. Retrieved July 28, 2022, from aeon.co/essays/blaming-individuals-for-obesity-may-be-altogether-wrong

Alexander, C. L. (2006). The emotional first + aid kit: A practical guide to life after bariatric surgery. Edgemont, PA: Matrix Medical Communications.

Altfas J. R. (2002). Prevalence of attention deficit/hyperactivity disorder among adults in obesity treatment. BMC psychiatry, 2, 9. doi.org/10.1186/1471-244x-2-9

Andersen, A. E. (1990). Males with eating disorders. Brunner/Mazel.

Andreyeva, T., Puhl, R. M. and Brownell, K. D. (2008), Changes in Perceived Weight Discrimination Among Americans, 1995–1996 Through 2004–2006. Obesity, 16: 1129–1134. doi:10.1038/oby.2008.35

Anorexia Nervosa. (2018, February 28). Retrieved October 21, 2020, from nationaleatingdisorders.org/learn/by-eating-disorder/anorexia

Arcelus, J., Mitchell, A. J., Wales, J., & Nielsen, S. (2011). Mortality rates in patients with Anorexia Nervosa and other eating disorders. Archives of General Psychiatry, 68(7), 724-731.

Are you a chronic self-abandoner? NAMI. (n.d.). Retrieved September 15, 2022, from nami.org/Blogs/NAMI-Blog/April-2018/Are-You-a-Chronic-Self-Abandoner

Austin, S. Bryn, Sc.D.. 2004. Sexual Orientation, Weight Concerns, and Eating- Disordered Behaviors in Adolescent Girls and Boys. Journal of the American Academy of Child & Adolescent Psychiatry, V43.

Avoidant Restrictive Food Intake Disorder (ARFID). (2018, February 22). Retrieved October 21, 2020, from nationaleatingdisorders.org/learn/by-eating-disorder/arfid

Becker, A. E., Franko, D. L., Speck, A., & Herzog, D. B. (2003). Ethnicity and differential access to care for eating disorder symptoms. International Journal of Eating Disorders, 33(2), 205-212. doi:10.1002/eat.10129

Bacon, L., Aphramor, L. Weight Science: Evaluating the Evidence for a Paradigm Shift. Nutr J 10, 9 (2011). doi.org/10.1186/1475-2891-10-9Beats, K. A., & Manore, M. M. (1999). Subclinical eating disorders in physically active women. *Topics in Clinical Nutrition*, 14(3), 14–29. doi.org/10.1097/00008486-199906000-00004

Biederman, J., Ball, S. W., Monuteaux, M. C., Surman, C. B., Johnson, J. L., & Zeitlin, S. (2007). Are girls with ADHD at risk for eating disorders? Results from a controlled, five-year prospective study. Journal of developmental and behavioral pediatrics : JDBP, 28(4), 302–307. doi.org/10.1097/DBP.0b013e3180327917

Bjork, C. (2020, April/May). How important is it to count calories and macros? I hate tracking everything I heat or drink. Is it really necessary to meet my goals? *Paleo Magazine*.

Bray, B., Rodríguez-Martín, B. C., Wiss, D. A., Bray, C. E., & Zwickey, H. (2021). Overeaters Anonymous: An Overlooked Intervention for Binge Eating Disorder. International journal of environmental research and public health, 18(14), 7303. doi.org/10.3390/ijerph18147303

Brennan, M. A., Lalonde, C. E., & Bain, J. L. (2010). Body image perceptions: Do gender differences exist? Psi Chi Journal of Psychological Research, 15(3), 130–138. doi.org/10.24839/1089-4136.jn15.3.130

Burlew, L. D., & Shurts, W. M. (2013). Men and body image: Current issues and counseling implications. *Journal of Counseling & Development*, 91(4), 428–435. doi.org/10.1002/j.1556-6676.2013.00114.x

Carlat, D.J., Camargo, CA, & Herzog, DB, 1991. Eating disorders in males: a report of 135 patients. American Journal of Psychiatry, 148, 1991.

Castonguay, A. L., Pila, E., Wrosch, C., & Sabiston, C. M. (2014). Body-related self-conscious emotions relate to physical activity motivation and behavior in men. *American Journal of Men's Health*, 9(3), 209–221. doi.org/10.1177/1557988314537517

Center for Disease Control and Massachusetts Department of Education. 1999. Massachusetts State Youth Risk Behavior Survey. National Gay and Lesbian Task Force (with National Coalition for the Homeless)

Chan, A. (2021, April 16). Lizzo feels the body-positivity movement has been 'co-opted by all bodies'. Billboard. Retrieved July 28, 2022, from billboard.com/music/music-news/lizzo-feels-body-positivity-movement-has-been-co-opted-9557044/

Chapa, D. A., Bohrer, B. K., & Forbush, K. T. (2018). Is the diagnostic threshold for bulimia nervosa clinically meaningful? *Eating Behaviors*, 28, 16-19. doi:10.1016/j.eatbeh.2017.12.002

Chard, C. A., Hilzendegen, C., Barthels, F., & Stroebele-Benschop, N. (2019). Psychometric evaluation of the English version of the Düsseldorf Orthorexie Scale (DOS) and the prevalence of orthorexia nervosa among a U.S. student sample. Eating and weight disorders : EWD, 24(2), 275–281. doi.org/10.1007/s40519-018-0570-6

Chen, J. (2020) Self-abandonment or seeking an alternative way out: understanding Chinese rural migrant children's resistance to schooling, British Journal of Sociology of Education, 41:2, 253-268, DOI: 10.1080/01425692.2019.1691504

Chesney, E., Goodwin, G. M., & Fazel, S. (2014). Risks of all-cause and suicide mortality in mental disorders: a meta-review. World Psychiatry, 13(2), 153-160.

Clients with substance use and eating disorders. (n.d.). Retrieved September 29, 2022, from store.samhsa.gov/sites/default/files/d7/priv/sma10-4617.pdf

Cohn, L. (2013). *Current findings on males with eating disorders*. Routledge.

Colori, S. (2015). Journaling as therapy. Schizophrenia Bulletin, 44(2), 226–228. doi.org/10.1093/schbul/sbv066

Compte, E.J., Cattle, C.J., Lavender, J.M. et al. Psychometric evaluation of the muscle dysmorphic disorder inventory (MDDI) among gender-expansive people. J Eat Disord 10, 95 (2022). doi.org/10.1186/s40337-022-00618-6

Conceição, E., Orcutt, M., Mitchell, J., Engel, S., Lahaise, K., Jorgensen, M., Woodbury, K., Hass, N., Garcia, L., & Wonderlich, S. (2013). Eating disorders after bariatric surgery: a case series. *The International journal of eating disorders*, 46(3), 274–279. doi.org/10.1002/eat.22074

Cordeiro, F., Epstein, D. A., Thomaz, E., Bales, E., Jagannathan, A. K., Abowd, G. D., & Fogarty, J. (2015). Barriers and negative nudges. Proceedings of the 33rd Annual ACM Conference on Human Factors in Computing Systems. doi.org/10.1145/2702123.2702155

Cortese, S., Moreira-Maia, C. R., St Fleur, D., Morcillo-Peñalver, C., Rohde, L. A., & Faraone, S. V. (2016). Association Between ADHD and Obesity: A Systematic Review and Meta-Analysis. The American journal of psychiatry, 173(1), 34–43. doi.org/10.1176/appi.ajp.2015.15020266

Counseling center. The University of Toledo. (n.d.). Retrieved October 26, 2022, from utoledo.edu/studentaffairs/counseling/selfhelp/substanceuse/marijuanatolerancewithdrawal.html

Cowden, S. (2020, February 18). Journaling topics for helping you recover from your eating disorder. Verywell Mind. Retrieved July 29, 2022, from verywellmind.com/journaling-topics-for-eating-disorders-1138293

Culbert, K. M., Racine, S. E., & Klump, K. L. (2015). Research Review: What we have learned about the causes of eating disorders —a synthesis of sociocultural, psychological, and biological research. J Child Psychol Psychiatry, 56(11), 1141-1164.

Cummings, J. R., Joyner, M. A., & Gearhardt, A. N. (2020). Development and preliminary validation of the Anticipated Effects of Food Scale. Psychology of addictive behaviors : journal of the Society of Psychologists in Addictive Behaviors, 34(2), 403–413. doi.org/10.1037/adb0000544

Curtin, C. , Pagoto, S. and Mick, E. (2013) The association between ADHD and eating disorders/pathology in adolescents: A systematic review. Open Journal of Epidemiology, 3, 193-202. doi: 10.4236/ojepi.2013.34028.

Daniel, S., & Bridges, S. K. (2013). The relationships among body image, masculinity, and sexual satisfaction in men. *Psychology of Men & Masculinity*, 14(4), 345–351. doi.org/10.1037/a0029154

Darcy, A. (2011). Eating disorders in adolescent males: An critical examination of five common assumptions. *Adolescent Psychiatry*, 1(4), 307–312. doi.org/10.2174/2210676611101040307

Devine, S., Germain, N., Ehrlich, S., & Eppinger, B. (2022). Changes in the Prevalence of Thin Bodies Bias Young Women's Judgments About Body Size. Psychological Science, 33(8), 1212–1225. doi.org/10.1177/09567976221082941

Diabulimia. National Eating Disorders Association. (2018, February 21). Retrieved September 27, 2022, from nationaleatingdisorders.org/diabulimia-5

Diemer, E. W., Grant, J. D., Munn-Chernoff, M. A., Patterson, D. A., & Duncan, A. E. (2015). Gender Identity, Sexual Orientation, and Eating-Related Pathology in a National Sample of College Students. Journal of Adolescent Health, 57(2), 144-149. doi:10.1016/j.jadohealth.2015.03.003

Eating Clay: Lessons from Worldwide Cultures. (2020, October 07). Retrieved October 21, 2020, from enviromedica.com/wellness/eating-clay-lessons-on-medicine-from-worldwide-cultures/

Eating disorders & athletes. National Eating Disorders Association. (2018, April 27). Retrieved September 29, 2022, from nationaleatingdisorders.org/eating-disorders-athletes

Eating disorders and autism. Eating Disorders Victoria. (2021, May 18). Retrieved August 18, 2022, from eatingdisorders.org.au/eating-disorders-a-z/eating-disorders-and-autism/

Eating Disorders vs. Disordered Eating: What's the Difference? (2018, February 21). Retrieved October 22, 2020, from nationaleatingdisorders.org/blog/eating-disorders-versus-disordered-eating

Eating healthy vs. unhealthy diet costs about $1.50 more per day. (2014, January 13). Retrieved March 18, 2021, from hsph.harvard.edu/news/press-releases/healthy-vs-unhealthy-diet-costs-1-50-more/

Fell, J. (2021, May 31). It's okay to want to lose weight. It's Okay to Want to Lose Weight. Retrieved July 28, 2022, from jamesfell.substack. com/p/its-okay-to-want-to-lose-weight?fbclid=IwAR1s4ZcMePEr ryEGJ8v8v-N2aHjoze-hG2rmpcRA-6KInmu70WewOF63Q54

Fell, J. (2019, July 25). Perhaps you should just stay fat. James Fell. Retrieved July 28, 2022, from bodyforwife.com/perhaps-you-should-just-stay-fat/

Fitzsimmons-Craft, E. E., Ciao, A. C., Accurso, E. C., Pisetsky, E. M., Peterson, C. B., Byrne, C. E., & Le Grange, D. (2014). Subjective and objective binge eating in relation to eating disorder symptomatology, depressive symptoms, and self-esteem among treatment-seeking adolescents with bulimia nervosa. *European eating disorders review : the journal of the Eating Disorders Association, 22*(4), 230–236. doi. org/10.1002/erv.2297

Fletcher, P.C., Kenny, P.J. Food addiction: a valid concept?. Neuropsychopharmacol *43*, 2506–2513 (2018). doi.org/10.1038/ s41386-018-0203-9

Forsén Mantilla E, Clinton D, Birgegård A. Insidious: The relationship patients have with their eating disorders and its impact on symptoms, duration of illness, and self-image. Psychol Psychother. 2018;91(3):302–316. doi:10.1111/papt.12161

Foroughi, A., Khanjani, S., & Mousavi Asl, E. (2019). Relationship of concern about body dysmorphia with external shame, perfectionism, and negative affect: The mediating role of self-compassion. Iranian Journal of Psychiatry and Behavioral Sciences, 13(2). doi.org/10.5812/ijpbs.80186

Franko, D. L., Dorer, D. J., Keel, P. K., Jackson, S., Manzo, M. P., & Herzog, D. B. (2005). How do eating disorders and alcohol use disorder influence each other? *International Journal of Eating Disorders, 38*(3), 200–207. doi.org/10.1002/eat.20178

Friend, Y. F. (2021, March 29). I'm a fat activist. here's why I don't use the word 'fatphobia'. SELF. Retrieved July 27, 2022, from self.com/ story/fat-activist-fatphobia

Galmiche, M., Déchelotte, P., Lambert, G., & Tavolacci, M. P. (2019). Prevalence of eating disorders over the 2000–2018 period: A Systematic Literature Review. The American Journal of Clinical Nutrition, 109(5), 1402–1413. doi.org/10.1093/ajcn/nqy342

Gaudiani, J. L. (2019). Sick enough: A guide to the medical complications of eating disorders. Routledge.

Gordon, D. F. (1984). Dying to self: Self-control through self-abandonment. Sociological Analysis, 45(1), 41. doi. org/10.2307/3711321

Gordon, E. L., Ariel-Donges, A. H., Bauman, V., & Merlo, L. J. (2018). What Is the Evidence for "Food Addiction?" A Systematic Review. Nutrients, 10(4), 477. doi.org/10.3390/nu10040477

Grange, D. L., Binford, R. B., Peterson, C. B., Crow, S. J., Crosby, R. D., Klein, M. H., . . . Wonderlich, S. A. (2006). DSM-IV threshold versus subthreshold bulimia nervosa. International Journal of Eating Disorders, 39(6), 462-467. doi:10.1002/eat.20304

Griffin, B.L., Vogt, K.S. Drunkorexia: is it really "just" a university lifestyle choice?. Eat Weight Disord 26, 2021–2031 (2021). doi. org/10.1007/s40519-020-01051-x

Grilo, C. M., White, M. A. and Masheb, R. M. (2009), DSM-IV psychiatric disorder comorbidity and its correlates in binge eating disorder. Int. J. Eat. Disord. 42: 228–234. doi:10.1002/eat.20599

Grunfeld C et al. Oxandrolone in the treatment of HIV-associated weight loss in men: a randomized, double-blind, placebo-controlled study. J Acquir Immune Defic Syndr 41: 304 – 314, 2006.

Golden, N. H., Schneider, M., & Wood, C. (2016). Preventing Obesity and Eating Disorders in Adolescents. Pediatrics, 138(3). doi:10.1542/peds.2016-1649

Goeree, Michelle Sovinsky, Ham, John C., & Iorio, Daniela. (2011). Race, Social Class, and Bulimia Nervosa. IZA Discussion Paper No. 5823. Retrieved from ftp.iza.org/dp5823.pdf.

Gudiksen, A., Qoqaj, A., Ringholm, S., Wojtaszewski, J., Plomgaard, P., & Pilegaard, H. (2021). Ameliorating effects of lifelong physical activity on healthy aging and mitochondrial function in human white adipose tissue. The Journals of Gerontology: Series A, 77(6), 1101–1111. doi.org/10.1093/gerona/glab356

Guillaume, S., Jaussent, I., Maimoun, L., Ryst, A., Seneque, M., Villain, L., Hamroun, D., Lefebvre, P., Renard, E., & Courtet, P. (2016). Associations between adverse childhood experiences and clinical characteristics of eating disorders. Scientific reports, 6, 35761. doi. org/10.1038/srep35761

Guerdjikova, A. I., & McElroy, S. L. (2013). Adjunctive Methylphenidate in the Treatment of Bulimia Nervosa Co-occurring with Bipolar Disorder and Substance Dependence. Innovations in clinical neuroscience, 10(2), 30–33.

Guss, C. E., Williams, D. N., Reisner, S. L., Austin, S. B., & Katz-Wise, S. L. (2017). Disordered weight management behaviors, nonprescription steroid use, and weight perception in transgender youth. *Journal of Adolescent Health*, *60*(1), 17–22. doi.org/10.1016/j.jadohealth.2016.08.027

Gutowski, K. A. (2013). Screening tools for body dysmorphic disorder in a cosmetic surgery setting. Yearbook of Plastic and Aesthetic Surgery, 2013, 71–72. doi.org/10.1016/j.yprs.2012.01.017

Harmon, K. (2010, July 28). Social ties Boost survival by 50 percent. Retrieved March 17, 2021, from scientificamerican.com/article/relationships-boost-survival/?redirect=1

Harrison PA, Beebe TJ, Park E. The Adolescent Health Review: a brief, multidimensional screening instrument. J Adolesc Health. 2001;29:131–139. [PubMed] [Google Scholar]

Hartmann, A. S., Rief, W., & Hilbert, A. (2012). Laboratory snack food intake, negative mood, and impulsivity in youth with ADHD symptoms and episodes of loss of control eating. Where is the missing link?. Appetite, 58(2), 672–678. doi.org/10.1016/j.appet.2012.01.006

Haynos, A. F., & Fruzzetti, A. E. (2015). Initial evaluation of a single-item screener to assess problematic dietary restriction. *Eating and weight disorders : EWD*, *20*(3), 405–413. doi.org/10.1007/s40519-014-0161-0

Health consequences. National Eating Disorders Association. (2018, February 22). Retrieved September 27, 2022, from nationaleatingdisorders.org/health-consequences

Hebebrand, J., Albayrak, Ö., Adan, R., Antel, J., Dieguez, C., de Jong, J., Leng, G., Menzies, J., Mercer, J. G., Murphy, M., van der Plasse, G., & Dickson, S. L. (2014). "eating addiction", rather than "Food addiction", better captures addictive-like eating behavior. Neuroscience & Biobehavioral Reviews, 47, 295–306. doi.org/10.1016/j.neubiorev.2014.08.016

Higginson, A. D., & McNamara, J. M. (2016). An adaptive response to uncertainty can lead to weight gain during dieting attempts. Evolution, medicine, and public health, 2016(1), 369–380. doi. org/10.1093/emph/eow031

Higginson, A. D., McNamara, J. M., & Houston, A. I. (2016). Fatness and fitness: exposing the logic of evolutionary explanations for obesity. Proceedings. Biological sciences, 283(1822), 20152443. doi. org/10.1098/rspb.2015.2443

Hobbes, M. (2018, September 19). Everything you know about obesity is wrong. Retrieved March 18, 2021, from highline.huffingtonpost. com/articles/en/everything-you-know-about-obesity-is-wrong/

Holtkamp, K., Konrad, K., Müller, B., Heussen, N., Herpertz, S., Herpertz-Dahlmann, B., & Hebebrand, J. (2004). Overweight and obesity in children with Attention-Deficit/Hyperactivity Disorder. International journal of obesity and related metabolic disorders : journal of the International Association for the Study of Obesity, 28(5), 685–689. doi.org/10.1038/sj.ijo.0802623

Hudson JI, Hiripi E, Pope HG Jr, and Kessler RC. (2007). The prevalence and correlates of eating disorders in the National Comorbidity Survey Replication. Biological Psychiatry, 61(3):348-58.

Insidious: The relationship patients have with ... —wiley online library. (n.d.). Retrieved July 21, 2022, from onlinelibrary.wiley.com/ doi/10.1111/papt.12161

Johnston, A. (2010). Eating in the light of the Moon how women can transform their relationships with food through myth, metaphors & storytelling. Gürze Books.

Hudson, J. I., Hiripi, E., Pope, H. G., Jr, & Kessler, R. C. (2007). The prevalence and correlates of eating disorders in the National Comorbidity Survey Replication. Biological psychiatry, 61(3), 348–358. doi.org/10.1016/j.biopsych.2006.03.040

Kain, J. (2018, May 30). Oryoki and eating just the right amount. Tricycle. Retrieved July 21, 2022, from tricycle.org/magazine/eating-just-right-amount/

Kaye WH, Bulik CM, Thornton L, Barbarich N, Masters K, "Comorbidity of anxiety disorders with anorexia and bulimia nervosa." Am J Psychiatry, 2004; 161 2215-2221. 2. Yaryura-Tobias JA, & Neziroglu

F (1983). "Obsessive Compulsive Disorders Pathogenesis Diagnosis and Treatment." New York Marcel Dekker

Klump KL, Bulik CK, Kaye W, Treasure J, Tyson E. Academy for Eating Disorders Position Paper: Eating Disorders are Serious Mental Illnesses. Int J Eat Disord. 2009 Mar;42(2):97-103. doi: 10.1002/eat.20589.

Knoll, J. (2019, June 08). Smash the wellness industry. Retrieved March 17, 2021, from nytimes.com/2019/06/08/opinion/sunday/women-dieting-wellness.html

Kusnik A, Vaqar S. Rumination Disorder. [Updated 2022 May 5]. In: StatPearls [Internet]. Treasure Island (FL): StatPearls Publishing; 2022 Jan-. Available from: ncbi.nlm.nih.gov/books/NBK576404/

Judkis, M. (2019, March 28). You might think there are more vegetarians than ever. you'd be wrong. Retrieved March 17, 2021, from washingtonpost.com/news/food/wp/2018/08/03/you-might-think-there-are-more-vegetarians-than-ever-youd-be-wrong/

Lawson, N. (2021, July 19). Nigella Lawson wants everyone to experience the (thoroughly guilt-free) pleasure of food. Literary Hub. Retrieved July 27, 2022, from lithub.com/nigella-lawson-wants-everyone-to-experience-the-thoroughly-guilt-free-pleasure-of-food/

Leptin: What it is, Function & Levels. Cleveland Clinic. (n.d.). Retrieved September 23, 2022, from my.clevelandclinic.org/health/articles/22446-leptin

Leone, J. E., Sedory, E. J., & Gray, K. A. (2005). Recognition and treatment of muscle dysmorphia and related body image disorders. Journal of athletic training, 40(4), 352–359.

Lien, C., Rosen, T., Bloemen, E. M., Abrams, R. C., Pavlou, M., & Lachs, M. S. (2016). Narratives of Self-Neglect: Patterns of Traumatic Personal Experiences and Maladaptive Behaviors in Cognitively Intact Older Adults. Journal of the American Geriatrics Society, 64(11), e195–e200. doi.org/10.1111/jgs.14524

Long C, G, Blundell J, E, Finlayson G: A Systematic Review of the Application And Correlates of YFAS-Diagnosed 'Food Addiction' in Humans: Are Eating-Related 'Addictions' a Cause for Concern or Empty Concepts? Obes Facts 2015;8:386-401. doi: 10.1159/000442403

Lydecker, J. A., Shea, M., & Grilo, C. M. (2017). Driven exercise in the absence of binge eating: Implications for purging disorder. International Journal of Eating Disorders, 51(2), 139–145. doi. org/10.1002/eat.22811

Lyons, P. (2009). Prescription for Harm: Diet Industry Influence, Public Health Policy, and the "Obesity Epidemic". In Wann M. (Author) & Rothblum E. & Solovay S. (Eds.), The Fat Studies Reader (pp. 75-87). NYU Press. Retrieved from jstor.org/stable/j.ctt9qg2bh.13

Malaeb, D., Bianchi, D., Pompili, S., Berro, J., Laghi, F., Azzi, V., Akel, M., Obeid, S., & Hallit, S. (2022). Drunkorexia behaviors and motives, eating attitudes and mental health in Lebanese alcohol drinkers: a path analysis model. Eating and weight disorders : EWD, 27(5), 1787–1797. doi.org/10.1007/s40519-021-01321-2

Mann, B., & Bebinger, M. (2022, March 3). Purdue Pharma, Sacklers reach $6 billion deal with state attorneys general. NPR. Retrieved September 23, 2022, from npr.org/2022/03/03/1084163626/ purdue-sacklers-oxycontin-settlement

Marques, L., Alegria, M., Becker, A. E., Chen, C., Fang, A., Chosak, A., & Diniz, J. B. (2011). Comparative Prevalence, Correlates of Impairment, and Service Utilization for Eating Disorders across U.S. Ethnic Groups: Implications for Reducing Ethnic Disparities in Health Care Access for Eating Disorders. The International Journal of Eating Disorders, 44(5), 412–420. doi.org/10.1002/eat.20787

Martin, S. (2018, December 21). Why we abandon ourselves and how to stop. Psych Central. Retrieved September 15, 2022, from psychcentral.com/blog/imperfect/2018/12/why-we-abandon-ourselves-and-how-to-stop#Why-we-abandon-ourselves

Mount R, Neziroglu F, Taylor CJ. "An obsessive-compulsive view of obesity and its treatment." J Clinical Psychology, Jan. 1990; 46 (1) 68-78.

Masur, L. (2019, June 27). The way we eat: Jessamyn Stanley, yoga teacher and activist in Durham, North Carolina. Kitchn. Retrieved July 29, 2022, from thekitchn.com/jessamyn-stanley-the-way-we-eat-267665

MAYES, HUMPHREY, HANDFORD, & MITCHELL, (1988). Rumination disorder: Differential diagnosis. Journal of the American Academy of Child & Adolescent Psychiatry, 27(3), 300–302. doi.org/10.1097/00004583-198805000-00006

Meinerding, M., Weinstock, J., Vander Wal, J., & Weaver, T. L. (2022). Failure to confirm the factor structure of the CEBRACS: An assessment of food and Alcohol Disturbance. Journal of American College Health, 1–11. doi.org/10.1080/07448481.2022.2119401

Migala, J. (2020, September). Food Worry Was Sapping My Energy. *Women's Health*.

Mikami, A. Y., Hinshaw, S. P., Patterson, K. A., & Lee, J. C. (2008). Eating pathology among adolescent girls with attention-deficit/hyperactivity disorder. Journal of abnormal psychology, 117(1), 225–235. doi.org/10.1037/0021-843X.117.1.225

Mitchison, D., Hay, P., Slewa-Younan, S., & Mond, J. (2014). The changing demographic profile of eating disorder behaviors in the community. *BMC public health*, *14*, 943. doi.org/10.1186/1471-2458-14-943

Mond, J.M., Mitchison, D., & Hay, P. (2014) "Prevalence and implications of eating disordered behavior in men" in Cohn, L., Lemberg, R. (2014) Current Findings on Males with Eating Disorders. Philadelphia, PA: Routledge.

Mond, J., Mitchison, D., Latner, J., Hay, P., Owen, C., & Rodgers, B. (2013). Quality of life impairment associated with body dissatisfaction in a general population sample of women. *BMC public health*, *13*, 920. doi.org/10.1186/1471-2458-13-920

Meule, A. & Gearhardt, A. (2019). Ten Years of the Yale Food Addiction Scale: a Review of Version 2.0. Current Addiction Reports. 10.1007/s40429-019-00261-3.

Meule, A., & Voderholzer, U. (2021). Orthorexia nervosa—it is time to think about abandoning the concept of a distinct diagnosis. Frontiers in Psychiatry, 12. doi.org/10.3389/fpsyt.2021.640401

Morgan, J. F., Reid, F., & Lacey, J. H. (1999). The Scoff Questionnaire: Assessment of a new screening tool for eating disorders. BMJ, 319(7223), 1467–1468. doi.org/10.1136/bmj.319.7223.1467

Muhlheim, L. (2021, February 28). How to identify purging disorder? Verywell Mind. Retrieved September 2, 2022, from verywellmind.com/purging-disorder-4157658

Munoz, L. (2019, June 21). Diet culture is more toxic than we realize—for all of us. Retrieved March 17, 2021, from greatist.com/live/toxic-diet-culture#6

Munzer, S. R. (2005). Self-abandonment and self-denial quietism, Calvinism, and the prospect of hell. Journal of Religious Ethics, 33(4), 747–781. doi.org/10.1111/j.1467-9795.2005.00246.x

Nazar, B. P., Bernardes, C., Peachey, G., Sergeant, J., Mattos, P., & Treasure, J. (2016). The risk of eating disorders comorbid with attention-deficit/hyperactivity disorder: A systematic review and meta-analysis. The International journal of eating disorders, 49(12), 1045–1057. doi.org/10.1002/eat.22643

Nicely, T. A., Lane-Loney, S., Masciulli, E., Hollenbeak, C. S., & Ornstein, R. M. (2014). Prevalence and characteristics of avoidant/restrictive food intake disorder in a cohort of young patients in day treatment for eating disorders. Journal of eating disorders, 2(1), 21. doi.org/10.1186/s40337-014-0021-3

Niedzielski, A., & Kaźmierczak-Wojtaś, N. (2021). Prevalence of orthorexia nervosa and its diagnostic tools—a literature review. International Journal of Environmental Research and Public Health, 18(10), 5488. doi.org/10.3390/ijerph18105488

Noakes T. D. (1987). Heart disease in marathon runners: a review. Medicine and science in sports and exercise, 19(3), 187-194.

Olivardia, R. (2022, September 24). ADHD and eating disorders: Research, diagnosis & treatment guidelines. ADDitude. Retrieved September 29, 2022, from additudemag.com/eating-disorders-adhd-research-treatments/?fbclid=IwAR0Fy-Mede5b7RLYb17yFqhkf7NcZUN1JGf6mf0hG_7rQ91yan7XNdo-OJA

Oosthuizen, P., Lambert, T., & Castle, D. J. (1998). Dysmorphic concern: prevalence and associations with clinical variables. Australian and New Zealand Journal of Psychiatry, 32(1), 129-132. doi: 10.3109/00048679809062719

Papadopoulos, F. C., A. Ekbom, L. Brandt, and L. Ekselius. "Excess Mortality, Causes of Death and Prognostic Factors in Anorexia Nervosa." The British Journal of Psychiatry 194.1 (2008): 10-17.

Parker-pope, T. (2007, December 05). A high price for healthy food. Retrieved March 18, 2021, from well.blogs.nytimes.com/2007/12/05/a-high-price-for-healthy-food/

Panduro A, Rivera-Iñiguez I, Sepulveda-Villegas M, Roman S. Genes, emotions and gut microbiota: The next frontier for the gastroenterologist. World J Gastroenterol. 2017;23(17):3030–3042. doi:10.3748/wjg.v23.i17.3030

Pica. (2018, February 22). Retrieved October 21, 2020, from nationaleatingdisorders.org/learn/by-eating-disorder/other/pica

Ptacek, R., Kuzelova, H., Stefano, G. B., Raboch, J., Sadkova, T., Goetz, M., & Kream, R. M. (2014). Disruptive patterns of eating behaviors and associated lifestyles in males with ADHD. Medical science monitor : international medical journal of experimental and clinical research, 20, 608–613. doi.org/10.12659/MSM.890495

Putnick, D. L., & Bornstein, M. H. (2016). Measurement Invariance Conventions and Reporting: The State of the Art and Future Directions for Psychological Research. Developmental review : DR, 41, 71–90. doi.org/10.1016/j.dr.2016.06.004

Recognizing and resisting diet culture. (2019, May 02). Retrieved March 18, 2021, from nationaleatingdisorders.org/blog/recognizing-and-resisting-diet-culture

Cohen, L., Rice, M., . . . Sacca, B. (2020, October 06). How influencers helped me dismantle Diet Culture. Retrieved March 18, 2021, from repeller.com/influencers-diet-culture/

Risk factors. National Eating Disorders Association. (2018, August 3). Retrieved August 18, 2022, from nationaleatingdisorders.org/risk-factors

Rothstein, C. (2020, January 21). The wellness industry isn't making you well. Retrieved March 17, 2021, from marieclaire.com/health-fitness/a23652473/wellness-industry-problems/

Rothblum, E. (2012-09-18). Fat Studies. Oxford Handbooks Online. Retrieved 8 May. 2017, from oxfordhandbooks.com/view/10.1093/oxfordhb/9780199736362.001.0001/oxfordhb-9780199736362-e-011.

Ruffle, J. K. (2014) Molecular neurobiology of addiction: what's all the (Δ)FosB about?, The American Journal of Drug and Alcohol Abuse, 40:6, 428-437, DOI: 10.3109/00952990.2014.933840

Rumination Disorder. (2018, February 22). Retrieved October 21, 2020, from nationaleatingdisorders.org/learn/by-eating-disorder/other/rumination-disorder

Rumination syndrome: Causes, signs & symptoms, treatment. Cleveland Clinic. (n.d.). Retrieved August 25, 2022, from my.clevelandclinic.org/health/diseases/17981-rumination-syndrome

Panduro, A., et al. Genes, emotions and gut microbiota: The Next Frontier for the gastroenterologist. World journal of gastroenterology. Retrieved July 21, 2022, from pubmed.ncbi.nlm. nih.gov/28533660/

Schulte, E. M., Smeal, J. K., Lewis, J., & Gearhardt, A. N. (2018). Development of the Highly Processed Food Withdrawal Scale. Appetite, 131, 148–154. doi.org/10.1016/j.appet.2018.09.013

Seitz, J., Kahraman-Lanzerath, B., Legenbauer, T., Sarrar, L., Herpertz, S., Salbach-Andrae, H., Konrad, K., & Herpertz-Dahlmann, B. (2013). The role of impulsivity, inattention and comorbid ADHD in patients with bulimia nervosa. PloS one, 8(5), e63891. doi. org/10.1371/journal.pone.0063891

Shaver, W. A. (2002). Suffering and the role of abandonment of self. Journal of Hospice & Palliative Nursing, 4(1), 46–53. doi. org/10.1097/00129191-200201000-00015

Smolak, L. (2011). Body image development in childhood. In T. Cash & L. Smolak (Eds.), Body Image: A Handbook of Science, Practice, and Prevention (2nd ed.).New York: Guilford.

Sport Nutrition for Coaches by Leslie Bonci, MPH, RD, CSSD, 2009, Human Kinetics. Byrne et al. 2001; Sundot—Borgen & Torstviet 2004

Stice E, Marti CN, Shaw H, and Jaconis M. (2010). An 8-year longitudinal study of the natural history of threshold, subthreshold, and partial eating disorders from a community sample of adolescents. Journal of Abnormal Psychology, 118(3):587-97. doi: 10.1037/a0016481.

Stice E, Cooper JA, Schoeller DA, Tappe K, Lowe MR. Are dietary restraint scales valid measures of moderate- to long-term dietary restriction? Objective biological and behavioral data suggest not. Psychol Assess. 2007;19:449–458. doi: 10.1037/1040-3590.19.4.449.

Stice, E., Rohde, P., Gau, J., & Shaw, H. (2009). An effectiveness trial of a dissonance-based eating disorder prevention program for high-risk adolescent girls. Journal of consulting and clinical psychology, 77(5), 825–834. doi.org/10.1037/a0016132

Striegel-Moore, R. H., Dohm, F. A., Solomon, E. E., Fairburn, C. G., Pike, K. M., & Wilfley, D. E. (2000). Subthreshold binge eating disorder. International Journal of Eating Disorders, 27(3), 270-278. doi:10.1002/(sici)1098-108x(200004)27:3.0.co;2-1

Sussex Publishers. (n.d.). *We are failing at treating eating disorders in minorities*. Psychology Today. Retrieved August 18, 2022, from psychologytoday.com/us/blog/happiness-is-state-mind/201902/we-are-failing-treating-eating-disorders-in-minorities

Swanson SA, Crow SJ, Le Grange D, Swendsen J, and Merikangas KR. (2011). Prevalence and correlates of eating disorders in adolescents. Results from the national comorbidity survey replication adolescent supplement. Archives of General Psychiatry, 68(7):714-23.

Sysko, R., Glasofer, D. R., Hildebrandt, T., Klimek, P., Mitchell, J. E., Berg, K. C., Peterson, C. B., Wonderlich, S. A., & Walsh, B. T. (2015). The eating disorder assessment for DSM-5 (EDA-5): Development and validation of a structured interview for feeding and eating disorders. The International journal of eating disorders, 48(5), 452–463. doi.org/10.1002/eat.22388

Tagay, S., Schlottbohm, E., Reyes-Rodriguez, M. L., Repic, N., & Senf, W. (2014). Eating disorders, trauma, PTSD, and psychosocial resources. Eating disorders, 22(1), 33-49.

Tagliabue, A., Ferraris, C., Martinelli, V., Pinelli, G., Repossi, I., & Trentani, C. (2012). Clinical and psychological features of normal-weight women with subthreshold anorexia nervosa: a pilot case-control observational study. *Neuro endocrinology letters*, *33*(5), 477–482.

Termorshuizen, J. D., Watson, H. J., Thornton, L. M., Borg, S., Flatt, R. E., MacDermod, C. M., Harper, L. E., Furth, E. F., Peat, C. M., & Bulik, C. M. (2020). Early impact of covid -19 on individuals with self-reported eating disorders: A survey of ~1,000 individuals in the United States and the Netherlands. International Journal of Eating Disorders, 53(11), 1780–1790. doi.org/10.1002/eat.23353

The health benefits of Healthy Body Fat. Feisty Menopause. (n.d.). Retrieved October 19, 2022, from feistymenopause.com/blog/bodyfat

The Ranch TN. (2014, January 12). Objective Binge Eating Vs. Subjective Binge Eating. Retrieved October 20, 2020, from recoveryranch.com/addiction-blog/objective-binge-eating-vs-subjective-binge-eating/

The National Center on Addiction and Substance Abuse (CASA) at Columbia University. Food for Thought: Substance Abuse and

Eating Disorders. The National Center on Addiction and Substance Abuse (CASA) Columbia University; New York: 2003.

Tiwari, P., Mishra, B. N., & Sangwan, N. S. (2014). Phytochemical and pharmacological properties of Gymnema sylvestre: an important medicinal plant. BioMed research international, 2014, 830285. doi.org/10.1155/2014/830285

Nicola Twilley, C. (2018, January 30). The ancient origins of dieting. Retrieved March 18, 2021, from theatlantic.com/health/archive/2018/01/the-ancient-origins-of-dieting/551828/

Vashi, N. A. (2016). *Obsession with perfection: Body dysmorphia.* Clinics in dermatology. Retrieved August 5, 2022, from pubmed.ncbi.nlm.nih.gov/27968940/

Wade, T. D., Keski-Rahkonen A., & Hudson J. (2011).Epidemiology of eating disorders. In M. Tsuang and M. Tohen (Eds.), Textbook in Psychiatric Epidemiology (3rd ed.) (pp. 343-360). New York: Wiley.

Wann, M. (2009). The Fat Studies Reader (Rothblum E. & Solovay S., Eds.). NYU Press. Retrieved from jstor.org/stable/j.ctt9qg2bh

What is self-abandonment? Center for Growth Therapy. (n.d.). Retrieved September 15, 2022, from thecenterforgrowth.com/tips/what-is-self-abandonment

Wellness is now a $4.2 trillion global industry. (2018, October 17). Retrieved March 17, 2021, from globalwellnessinstitute.org/pressroom/press-releases/wellness-now-a-4-2-trillion-global-industry/

Westerberg, D. P., & Waitz, M. (2013). Binge-eating disorder. Osteopathic Family Physician, 5(6), 230-233.

Wooding, S. . (2022, September 13). A taste for sweet – an anthropologist explains the evolutionary origins of why you're programmed to Love sugar. The Conversation. Retrieved September 20, 2022, from theconversation.com/a-taste-for-sweet-an-anthropologist-explains-the-evolutionary-origins-of-why-youre-programmed-to-love-sugar-173197

Yo-yo dieting may increase women's heart disease risk. (n.d.). Retrieved March 17, 2021, from newsroom.heart.org/news/yo-yo-dieting-may-increase-womens-heart-disease-risk

More by Dr. Faith

Books
The Autism Relationships Handbook (with Joe Biel)
Coping Skills
How to Be Accountable (with Joe Biel)
This Is Your Brain on Depression
Unfuck Your Addiction
Unfuck Your Adulting
Unfuck Your Anger
Unfuck Your Anxiety
Unfuck Your Blow Jobs
Unfuck Your Body
Unfuck Your Boundaries
Unfuck Your Brain
Unfuck Your Cunnilingus
Unfuck Your Grief
Unfuck Your Friendships
Unfuck Your Intimacy
Unfuck Your Sex Toys
Unfuck Your Worth
Unfuck Your Writing (with Joe Biel)
Woke Parenting (with Bonnie Scott)

Workbooks
Achieve Your Goals
The Autism Relationships Workbook (with Joe Biel)
How to Be Accountable Workbook (with Joe Biel)
Unfuck Your Anger Workbook
Unfuck Your Anxiety Workbook
Unfuck Your Body Workbook
Unfuck Your Boundaries Workbook
Unfuck Your Intimacy Workbook
Unfuck Your Worth Workbook
Unfuck Your Year

Other
Boundaries Conversation Deck
How Do You Feel Today? (poster)
Zines
The Autism Handbook (with Joe Biel)
The Autism Partner Handbook (with Joe Biel)
BDSM FAQ
Dating
Defriending
Detox Your Masculinity (with Aaron Sapp)
Emotional Freedom Technique
The Five Emotional Hungers
Getting Over It
How to Find a Therapist
How to Say No
Indigenous Noms
Relationshipping
The Revolution Won't Forget the Holidays
Self-Compassion
Sex Tools
Sexing Yourself
STI FAQ (with Aaron Sapp)
Surviving
This Is Your Brain on Addiction
This Is Your Brain on Grief
This Is Your Brain on PTSD
Unfuck Your Consent
Unfuck Your Forgiveness
Unfuck Your Mental Health Paradigm
Unfuck Your Sleep
Unfuck Your Stress
Unfuck Your Work
Vision Boarding
Woke Parenting #1-6 (with Bonnie Scott)

ABOUT THE AUTHOR

Faith Harper PhD, LPC-S, ACS, ACN is a bad-ass, funny lady with a PhD. She's a licensed professional counselor, board supervisor, certified sexologist, and applied clinical nutritionist with a private practice and consulting business in San Antonio, TX. She has been an adjunct professor and a TEDx presenter, and proudly identifies as a woman of color and uppity intersectional feminist. She is the author of dozens of books.

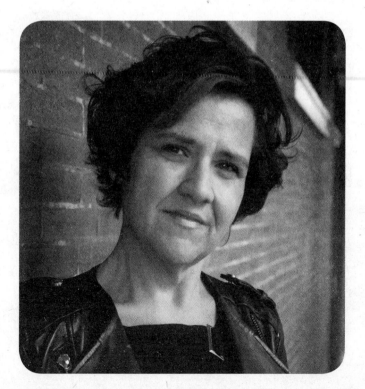

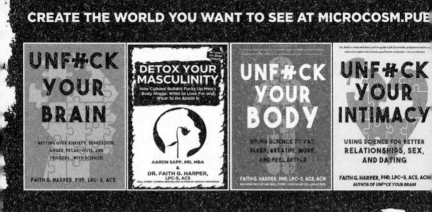

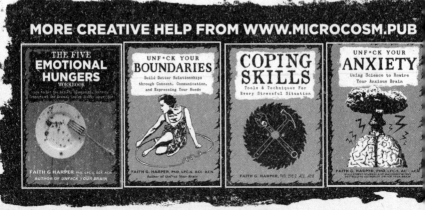